Taylor and Kelly's
Color Atlas and Synopsis
for Skin of Color

T0091703

Taylor and Elbuluk's
Color Atlas and Synopsis for Skin of Color

Susan C. Taylor, MD
Bernett L. Johnson Endowed Professor
Director, Skin of Color Research Fellowship
Vice Chair for Diversity, Equity and Inclusion, Department of Dermatology
Perelman School of Medicine at the University of Pennsylvania
Past Vice-President American Academy of Dermatology (2020-2021)
Founder, Skin of Color Society
Philadelphia, Pennsylvania

Nada M. Elbuluk, MD, MSc
Associate Professor of Clinical Dermatology
Director, Skin of Color & Pigmentary Disorders Program
Director, Skin of Color Research Fellowship
Director, Dermatology Diversity & Inclusion Program
USC Department of Dermatology, Keck School of Medicine
Department of Dermatology
Keck School of Medicine
University of Southern California
Los Angeles, California

New York   Chicago   San Francisco   Athens   London   Madrid   Mexico City
Milan   New Delhi   Singapore   Sydney   Toronto

1 2 3 4 5 6 7   DSS   26 25 24 23

ISBN 978-1-264-26890-0
MHID 1-264-26890-4

This book was set in Myriad Pro by KnowledgeWorks Global Ltd.
The editors were Dimana Tzvetkova and Kim J. Davis.
The production supervisor was Richard Ruzycka.
Project management was provided by Revathi Viswanathan of KnowledgeWorks Global Ltd.
The designer was Mary McKeon.
The cover designer was W2 Design.

This book is printed on acid-free paper.

Library of Congress Cataloging-in-Publication Data

Names: Taylor, Susan C., author. | Elbuluk, Nada M., author.
Title: Taylor and Elbuluk's color atlas and synopsis for skin of color /
   Susan C. Taylor, Nada M. Elbuluk.
Other titles: Color atlas and synopsis for skin of color
Description: New York : McGraw Hill, [2023] | Includes index. | Summary:
   "This book provides a comparative study of dermatologic problems in skin
   of color"— Provided by publisher.
Identifiers: LCCN 2022014722 (print) | LCCN 2022014723 (ebook) | ISBN
   9781264268900 (paperback : alk. paper) | ISBN 9781264268917 (ebook)
Subjects: MESH: Skin Diseases | Ethnicity | Skin Pigmentation
Classification: LCC RL73.3 (print) | LCC RL73.3 (ebook) | NLM WR 140 |
   DDC 616.50089—dc23/eng/20220727
LC record available at https://lccn.loc.gov/2022014722
LC ebook record available at https://lccn.loc.gov/2022014723

McGraw Hill books are available at special quantity discounts to use as premiums and sales promotions or for use in corporate training programs. To contact a representative, please visit the Contact Us pages at www.mhprofessional.com.

Contents

Preface .... *vii*
Acknowledgments .... *ix*

SECTION 1: Normal Skin Variants 1
  1. Normal Variants in Pigmented Skin 3

SECTION 2: Inflammatory/Papulosquamous Disorders 9
  2. Atopic Dermatitis 11
  3. Psoriasis 29
  4. Contact Dermatitis 49
  5. Pityriasis Lichenoides Chronica 61
  6. Pityriasis Rosea 65
  7. Seborrheic Dermatitis 71
  8. Lichen Planus 77
  9. Lichen Nitidus 89

SECTION 3: Infections 93
  10. Tinea Versicolor 95
  11. Tinea Corporis 101
  12. Cellulitis 107
  13. Syphilis 111
  14. Verruca 117
  15. Molluscum 123
  16. Herpes Simplex and Varicella Zoster 127
  17. Scabies 133
  18. Erythema Chronicum Migrans 139

SECTION 4: Follicular Disorders 141
  19. Acne 143
  20. Rosacea 151
  21. Perioral Dermatitis 157
  22. Folliculitis 161
  23. Hidradenitis Suppurativa 167
  24. Pseudofolliculitis Barbae 171
  25. Acne Keloidalis Nuchae 177

SECTION 5: Benign Neoplasms 181
26. Dermatosis Papulosis Nigra and Seborrheic Keratoses 183
27. Dermatofibroma and Dermatofibroma Sarcoma Protuberans 187
28. Keloids and Hypertrophic Scars 195

SECTION 6: Malignancies 199
29. Basal Cell Carcinoma...201
30. Squamous Cell Carcinoma...207
31. Melanoma...213
32. Cutaneous T-Cell Lymphoma...219

SECTION 7: Pigmentary Disorders.. 227
33. Melanonychia...229
34. Melasma..233
35. Postinflammatory Pigment Alteration 239

SECTION 8: Photosensitive Disorders 247
36. Polymorphous Light Eruption..249
37. Chronic Actinic Dermatitis...255

SECTION 9: Drug Reactions 259
38. Morbilliform Drug Reactions 261
39. Fixed Drug Reactions...265
40. Stevens-Johnson Syndrome and Toxic Epidermal
    Necrolysis..269
41. Erythema Multiforme 273

SECTION 10: Common Cutaneous Disorders in Skin of
            Color Populations... 275
42. Sarcoidosis..277
43. Discoid Lupus Erythematosus/Chronic Cutaneous Lupus
    Erythematosus...285
44. Vasculitis...289
45. Cutaneous Manifestations of Diabetes Mellitus 293

SECTION 11: Benign Skin Findings 297
46. Striae Distensae...299
47. Extrinsic Aging 301

    Index *311*

Preface

We are honored and delighted to present *Taylor and Elbuluk's Color Atlas and Synopsis for Skin of Color*, which serves as a companion to the comprehensive textbook, *Taylor and Kelly's Dermatology for Skin of Color*. *Taylor and Elbuluk's Color Atlas and Synopsis for Skin of Color*, with over 350 photographs, is designed to serve as a comprehensive visual atlas to educate medical students, residents, attending physicians, and other healthcare providers to recognize common cutaneous disorders in patients with dark compared to white skin. Through images and in-depth descriptions, the book compares and contrasts unique differences in location and morphology of common skin disorders in skin of color compared to white skin.

There is a well-recognized dearth of dermatologic images of cutaneous diseases in patients with skin of color. This disparity is observed in medical student curricular and board preparation resources, textbooks, lectures, and online web-based medical resources. Medical students evaluated on their ability to recognize skin disease in lighter versus darker skin types (Fitzpatrick I–III versus Fitzpatrick IV–VI phototypes) demonstrated that they were less accurate in identifying common conditions in darker skin types. However, all medical students should be able to recognize common skin disorders in skin of color patients—knowledge that will serve them and their patients well in any medical specialty they choose.

Textbooks for dermatology trainees depict skin disorders primarily on white skin. One study demonstrated an average of only 19.5% skin of color images across six textbooks and two web-based resources geared toward dermatology residents. Regarding exposure of dermatologists to skin of color images, again, as with textbooks, there are insufficient images in conference sessions, dermatology continuing medical education programs, and dermatology journals.

The population of the United States, as well as worldwide, continues to become more diverse with each passing year. Dermatologists will be increasingly tasked with identifying disease in darker skin types and distinguishing normal from pathologic signs. The ability to accurately do so will be essential in the journey to improving healthcare outcomes and achieving heath equity for all. *Taylor and Elbuluk's Color Atlas and Synopsis for Skin of Color* will undoubtedly serve as an invaluable tool to assist dermatologists and the medical community in identifying disorders in skin of color populations.

Susan C. Taylor, MD
Nada M. Elbuluk, MD, MSc

Acknowledgments

"Of all the forms of inequality, injustice in health care is the most shocking and inhumane."

This profound quote from Martin Luther King, Jr., is the motivation for writing *Taylor and Kelly's Dermatology for Skin of Color* and now the companion, *Taylor and Elbuluk's Color Atlas and Synopsis for Skin of Color*. These two comprehensive books will allow dermatologists, residents, medical students, and other healthcare providers to recognize, diagnose, and treat dermatologic disorders in patients with skin of color and address health disparities in dermatology.

To my husband, Kemel Dawkins, and my daughters, Morgan Elizabeth and Madison Lauren, thank you for your love and support. You make all of my projects possible.

To my co-author, Nada Elbuluk, you have been such a pleasure to work with and have provided keen insight into the organization and execution of the *Atlas*. Thank you also for your determination to complete this project despite many early mornings. I am proud to have you as a colleague.

To the team at McGraw Hill, we thank you for sharing our vision for the *Atlas*. We particularly thank our editorial team for their guidance throughout the entire process. Additionally, we would like to thank Yacine Sow for her contributions to image acquisition.

Susan C. Taylor, MD

To my parents, Malik and Fadwa, and my grandparents, I am forever indebted to you. Thank you for sacrificing everything for your children to have the opportunities they have and supporting us in our personal and professional journeys. I would not be where I am without you.

To my husband, Jason, and our daughters, Laila and Mimi, you are the light of my life. Thank you for believing in me and making me feel that with your love and support anything is possible.

To Dr. Susan Taylor, thank you for this opportunity to work together on such an important contribution to the medical literature. It has been a beautiful and educational journey that I will always cherish. Beyond that, thank you for your mentorship, your support, your friendship, and for all you have done for our specialty. Your leadership and contributions have shaped an incredible legacy.

To my mentors—though there are too many to name, I want to thank a few of my closest mentors who have been with me since my early days as a medical student and resident. To Dr. Sewon Kang, Dr. William James, Dr. Pearl Grimes, and Dr. Amit Pandya, thank you isn't enough for the time and belief you invested in me and for the ways in which you each shaped my growth and professional career. I stand on your shoulders and thank you for supporting me then and now.

To the McGraw Hill team, thank you for your support of this important work through which we hope to improve health equity.

Nada M. Elbuluk, MD, MSc

Taylor and Elbuluk's
Color Atlas and Synopsis
for Skin of Color

Normal Skin Variants

CHAPTER 1 ▪ NORMAL VARIANTS IN PIGMENTED SKIN

KEY POINTS

- Pigmented skin can have alterations in pigmentation that can be considered normal variants.

- These include mucosal as well as palmar and plantar macular pigmentation.

- Nail plates may have vertical streaks of pigmentation.

- Bony prominences such as elbows and knees can also have generalized darkening.

- Embryologic lines of development can also lead to differences in the color of the dorsal versus ventral surfaces of the skin.

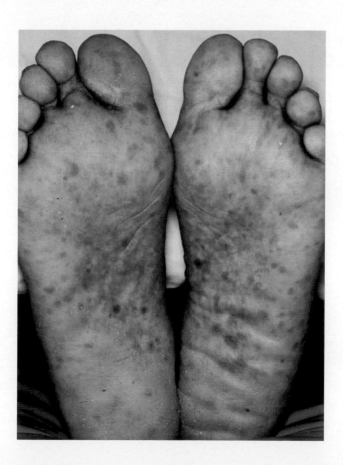

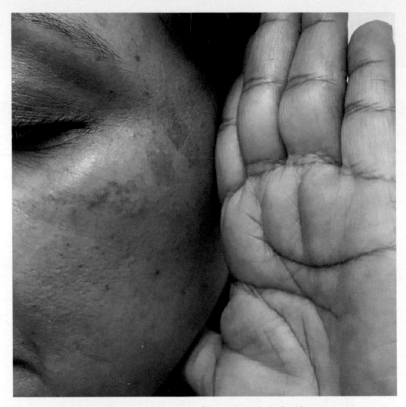

FIGURE 1-1. Brown linear creases on the palm of a person with darker skin. (Reproduced with permission from Leal-Silva H. Predicting the risk of postinflammatory hyperpigmentation: The palmar creases pigmentation scale. *J Cosmet Dermatol.* 2021;20(4):1263-1270.)

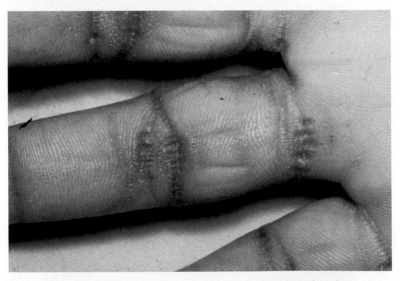

FIGURE 1-2. Atrophic brown punctate keratoses presenting linearly in the palmar creases of the digits. (Reproduced with permission from Taylor SC, Kelly AP, Lim HW, et al. *Taylor and Kelly's Dermatology for Skin of Color*, 2nd ed. New York, NY: McGraw Hill; 2016, Figure 20-9C.)

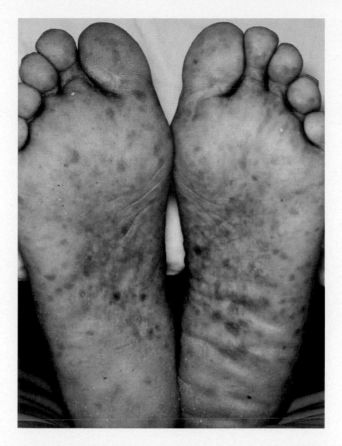

FIGURE 1-3. Numerous bilateral light to dark brown macules scattered on the plantar feet. (Reproduced with permission from Taylor SC, Kelly AP, Lim HW, et al. *Taylor and Kelly's Dermatology for Skin of Color*, 2nd ed. New York, NY: McGraw Hill; 2016, Figure 20-9A.)

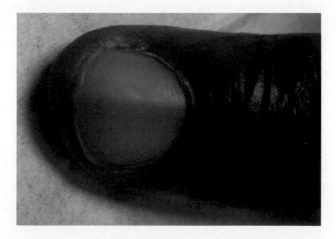

FIGURE 1-4. Faint light brown linear vertical streak on the nail plate of a person with darker skin. (Reproduced with permission from Taylor SC, Kelly AP, Lim HW, et al. *Taylor and Kelly's Dermatology for Skin of Color*, 2nd ed. New York, NY: McGraw Hill; 2016, Figure 21-3.)

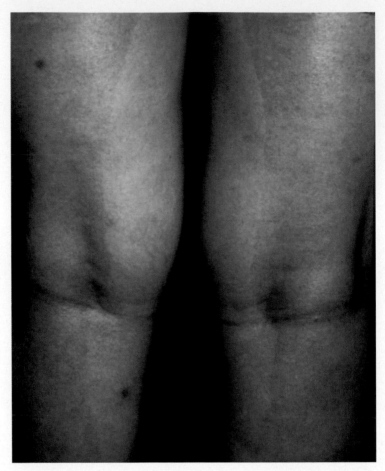

FIGURE 1-5. Sharp linear demarcation of pigmentation on the posterior lower extremities with darker brown skin laterally and lighter skin medially consistent with type B pigmentary demarcation lines also known as Futcher lines. (Reproduced with permission from Burgin S. *Guidebook to Dermatologic Diagnosis.* New York, NY: McGraw Hill; 2021, Figure 1-6D.)

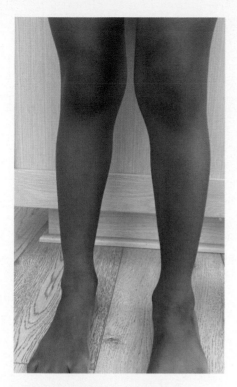

FIGURE 1-6. Increased pigmentation of the bilateral knees contrasting with the baseline skin color seen on the shins and dorsal feet. This is normal variant darkening, which can be seen in many individuals of color.

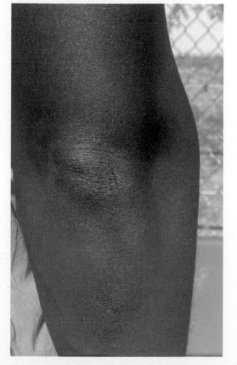

FIGURE 1-7. Darkening of the extensor elbow, a normal variant that can be seen in darker skin.

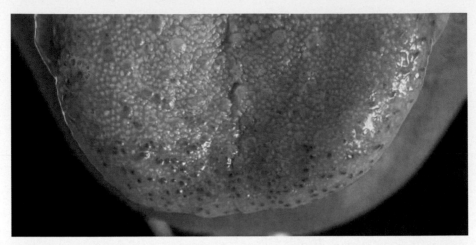

FIGURE 1-8. Medium brown pinpoint macules on the distal tongue, which can be present as a normal variant in individuals with pigmented skin.

Inflammatory/ Papulosquamous Disorders

KEY POINTS

- Active and chronic presentations of atopic dermatitis can differ in color and morphology in lighter and darker skin.

- Active disease in lighter skin can often present with patches and plaques that are pink to red and erythematous compared to brown to violaceous in darker skin.

- Morphology in darker skin can include follicular and papular presentations compared to patch and plaque morphology seen in lighter skin.

- Chronic disease in darker skin can also present with postinflammatory pigment change.

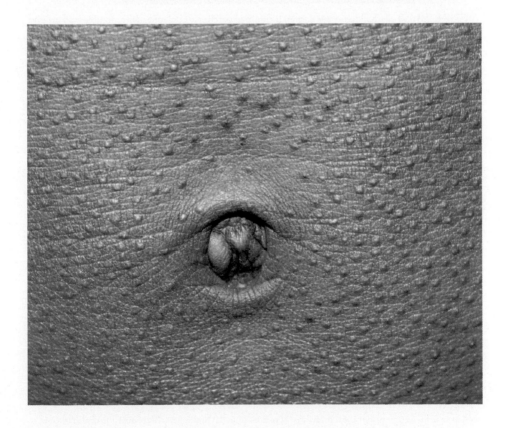

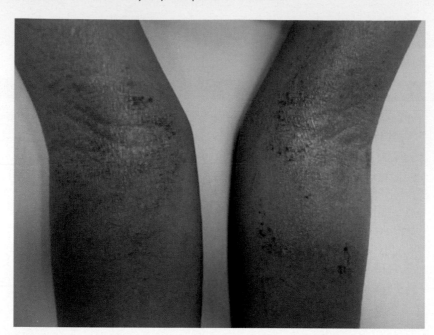

FIGURE 2-1. Ill-defined hyperpigmented lichenified patches and plaques with notable background erythema and overlying scale and excoriations. Fine papules representing follicular accentuation are noted above and below the antecubital fossa. Hypopigmented macules can also be seen peripherally on both extremities. (Reproduced with permission from Kane KS, Nambudiri VE, Stratigos AJ. *Color Atlas & Synopsis of Pediatric Dermatology*, 3rd ed. New York, NY: McGraw Hill; 2017, Figure 2-5.)

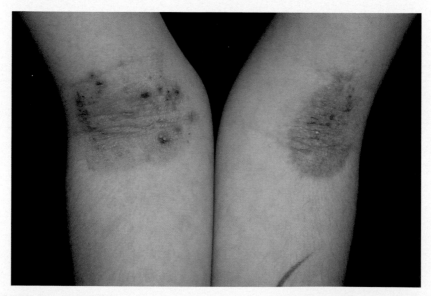

FIGURE 2-2. Well-defined, nummular, erythematous lichenified plaques with overlying scale as well as central and peripheral excoriations. (From Usatine RP, Smith MA, Mayeaux EJ Jr, et al. *The Color Atlas and Synopsis of Family Medicine*, 3rd ed. New York, NY: McGraw Hill; 2019. Figure 151-9. Reproduced with permission from Richard P. Usatine, MD.)

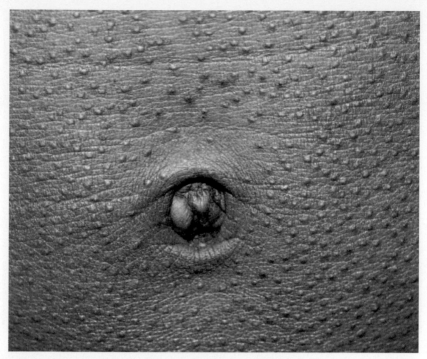

FIGURE 2-3. Periumbilical follicular accentuation represented by pinpoint skin-colored and hyperpigmented papules. (Reproduced with permission from Prose NS, Kristal L. *Weinberg's Color Atlas of Pediatric Dermatology*, 5th ed. New York, NY: McGraw Hill; 2017, Figure 9-22.)

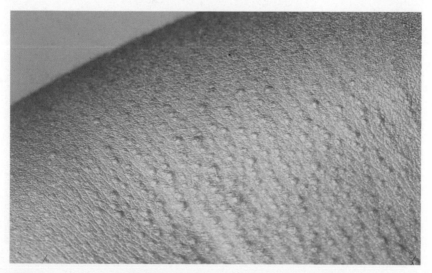

FIGURE 2-4. Close-up image highlighting pinpoint papules representing follicular accentuation along lines of cleavage, which are the same as the person's baseline skin color. (Reproduced with permission from Taylor SC, Kelly AP, Lim HW, et al. *Taylor and Kelly's Dermatology for Skin of Color*, 2nd ed. New York, NY: McGraw Hill; 2016, Figure 21-10.)

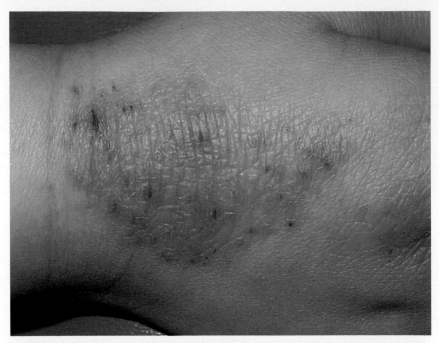

FIGURE 2-5. Nummular, pink, lichenified plaque with linear excoriations along cleavage lines. (Reproduced with permission from Soutor C, Hordinsky MK. *Clinical Dermatology.* New York, NY: McGraw Hill; 2013, Figure 2-10.)

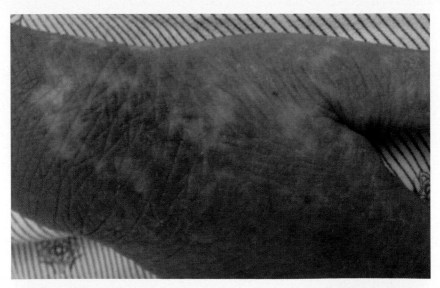

FIGURE 2-6. Diffuse lichenification of hyperpigmented and pink hypopigmented patches with fine overlying scale consistent with chronic atopic dermatitis. (Reproduced with permission from Taylor SC, Kelly AP, Lim HW, et al. *Taylor and Kelly's Dermatology for Skin of Color,* 2nd ed. New York, NY: McGraw Hill; 2016, Figure 85-4.)

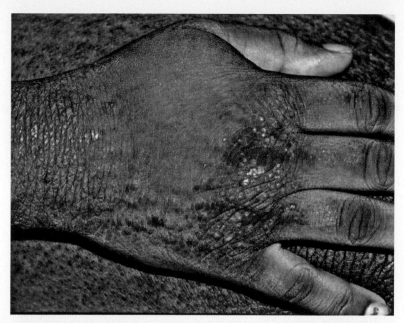

FIGURE 2-7. Confluent hyperpigmented lichenified papules along the lines of cleavage coalescing into hyperpigmented plaques on the extensor wrist and metacarpophalangeal joints. Note the background xerosis and chronic changes of atopic dermatitis along the lateral first and fifth digits. Pinpoint hyperpigmented papules can also be seen between the distal interphalangeal and metacarpophalangeal joints. Active disease is evidenced by fine papules along the metacarpophalanageal joints and dorsal digits. (Reproduced with permission from Prose NS, Kristal L. *Weinberg's Color Atlas of Pediatric Dermatology*, 5th ed. New York, NY: McGraw Hill; 2017, Figure 9-13.)

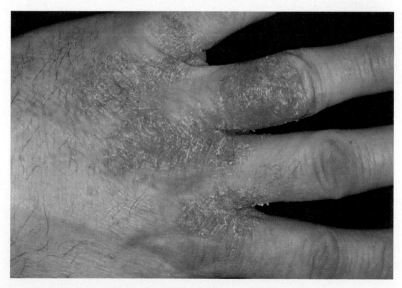

FIGURE 2-8. Pink scaly lichenified patches and plaques on the dorsal hand. (Reproduced with permission from Habif TP. *Clinical Dermatology: A Color Guide to Diagnosis and Therapy.* St. Louis, MO: Elsevier; 2016.)

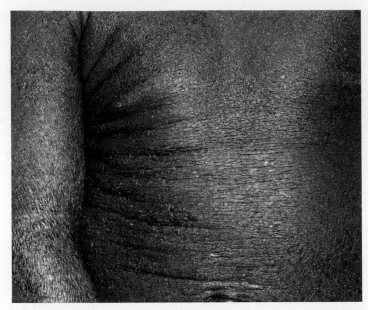

FIGURE 2-9. Diffuse, confluent, hyperpigmented, and lichenified scaly patch and plaques representative of chronic disease changes. Note the hyperpigmented fine papules along the bottom right corner of the figure. The central abdomen is notable for clustered dark-brown scabs. Linear pink erythema also can be seen in the antecubital fossa, signifying active disease. (Reproduced with permission from Prose NS, Kristal L. *Weinberg's Color Atlas of Pediatric Dermatology*, 5th ed. New York, NY: McGraw Hill; 2017, Figure 9-14.)

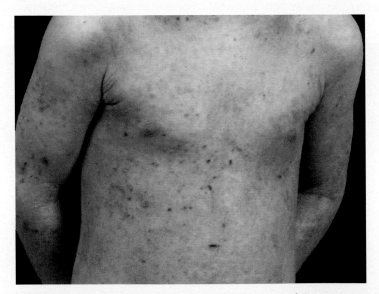

FIGURE 2-10. Diffuse erythematous and red papules and plaques overlying numerous pink patches interspersed with normal skin. Bilaterally on the ventral upper extremities are chronic changes of atopic dermatitis represented by erythematous lichenified plaques. (Reproduced with permission from Wolff K, Johnson RA, Saavedra AP, et al. *Fitzpatrick's Color Atlas and Synopsis of Clinical Dermatology*, 8th ed. New York, NY: McGraw Hill; 2017, Figure 2-15A.)

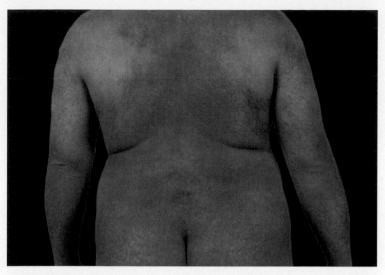

FIGURE 2-11. Diffuse hyperpigmented patches extending from the upper mid-back to the buttocks. Note the scaling and background xerosis bilateral to the gluteal cleft. (Reproduced with permission from Wolff K, Johnson RA, Saavedra AP, et al. *Fitzpatrick's Color Atlas and Synopsis of Clinical Dermatology*, 8th ed. New York, NY: McGraw Hill; 2017, Figure 2-15B.)

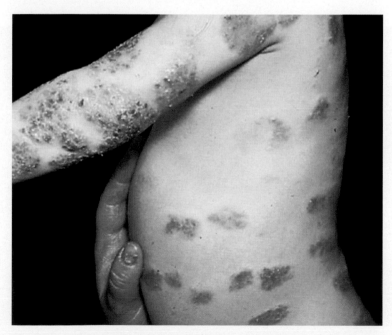

FIGURE 2-12. Numerous scattered, nummular, bright-red erythematous plaques with overlying scaling, excoriations, and impetiginization on a background of normal-appearing skin. Inferior to the axilla is also a dusky patch representing postinflammatory erythema secondary to resolving atopic dermatitis. (Reproduced with permission from Prose NS, Kristal L. *Weinberg's Color Atlas of Pediatric Dermatology*, 5th ed. New York, NY: McGraw Hill; 2017, Figure 9-11.)

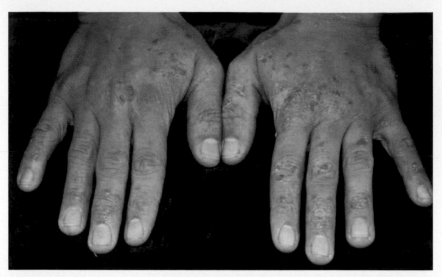

FIGURE 2-13. Dorsal hands of a Middle Eastern person with psoriasiform-like, pink-red lichenified plaques varying in size and scattered over the dorsal digits, metacarpophalangeal joints, and dorsal hands without coexisting pigmentary change. (Reproduced with permission from Taylor SC, Kelly AP, Lim HW, et al. *Taylor and Kelly's Dermatology for Skin of Color*, 2nd ed. New York, NY: McGraw Hill; 2016, Figure 92-3.)

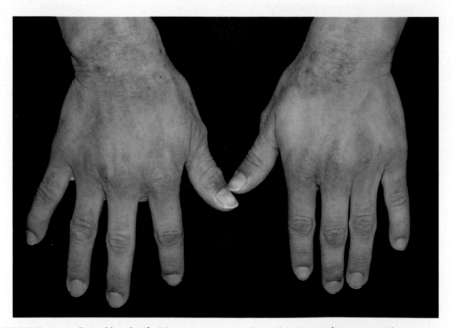

FIGURE 2-14. Dorsal hands of a Hispanic woman with overlapping erythematous and hyperpigmented lichenified patches and plaques on the extensor wrist and dorsal metacarpophalangeal joints. A few overlying papules are visible along cleavage lines as well as a few scattered excoriations. (From Usatine RP, Smith MA, Mayeaux EJ Jr, et al. *The Color Atlas and Synopsis of Family Medicine*, 3rd ed. New York, NY: McGraw Hill; 2019, Figure 153-11. Reproduced with permission from Richard P. Usatine, MD.)

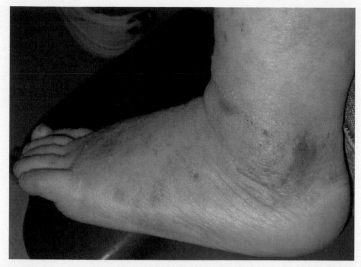

FIGURE 2-15. Pink lichenified patches and plaques with overlying excoriations on the left dorsal digits, foot, and extending onto the lateral ankle and lower extremity, with sparing of the transgrediens. (From Usatine RP, Smith MA, Mayeaux EJ Jr, et al. *The Color Atlas and Synopsis of Family Medicine*, 3rd ed. New York, NY: McGraw Hill; 2019, Figure 151-12. Reproduced with permission from Richard P. Usatine, MD.)

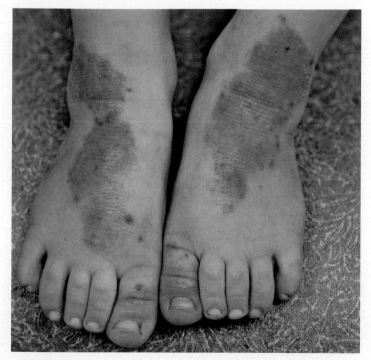

FIGURE 2-16. Bilateral, symmetric, well-demarcated, lichenified, pink-red plaques on dorsal feet extending onto the anterior ankles and toes. Note the overlying scattered peripheral red papules and linear erythema on the dorsal toes. (Reproduced with permission from Prose NS, Kristal L. *Weinberg's Color Atlas of Pediatric Dermatology*, 5th ed. New York, NY: McGraw Hill; 2017, Figure 9-12.)

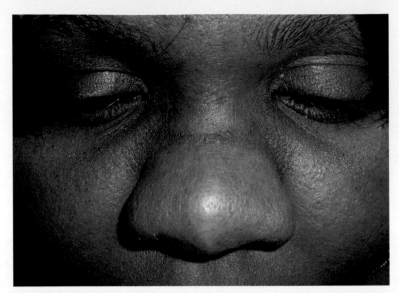

FIGURE 2-17. Periorbital edema with eyelid hyperpigmentation as well as notable allergic salute signified by hyperpigmented horizontal nasal crease extending onto the medial cheeks. (From Usatine RP, Smith MA, Mayeaux EJ Jr, et al. *The Color Atlas and Synopsis of Family Medicine*, 3rd ed. New York, NY: McGraw Hill; 2019, Figure 151-21. Reproduced with permission from Richard P. Usatine, MD.)

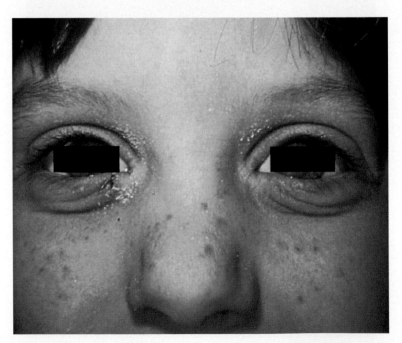

FIGURE 2-18. Bilateral periorbital edema of the upper and lower eyelids with Dennie–Morgan lines and overlying scaling and crusting on the medial eyelids. (Reproduced with permission from Prose NS, Kristal L. *Weinberg's Color Atlas of Pediatric Dermatology*, 5th ed. New York, NY: McGraw Hill; 2017, Figure 9-7.)

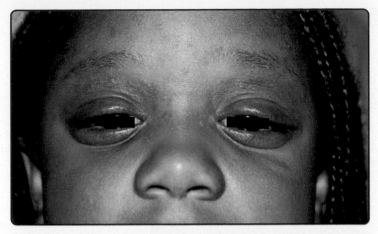

FIGURE 2-19. Bilateral periorbital edema of the upper and lower eyelids with Dennie–Morgan lines and diffuse ill-defined hyperpigmentation and lichenification of the eyelids, with fine papules clustered along the superior upper eyelids. (Reproduced with permission from Kang S, Amagai M, Bruckner AL, et al. *Fitzpatrick's Dermatology*, 9th ed. New York, NY: McGraw Hill; 2019, Figure 22-2.)

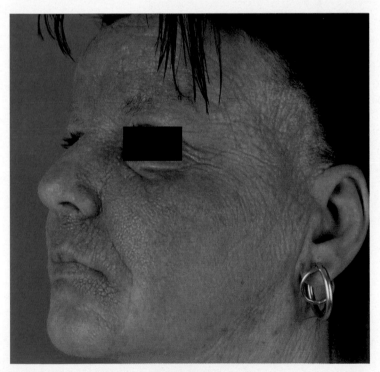

FIGURE 2-20. Diffuse background erythema with increased redness on the central face. Also notable is the diffuse lichenification, lateral excoriations along the jawline and earlobe, and Dennie–Morgan lines, as well as the thickening of the central facial skin resembling leonine facies. These changes represent an acute flare of severe chronic atopic dermatitis. (Reproduced with permission from Wolff K, Johnson RA, Saavedra AP, et al. *Fitzpatrick's Color Atlas and Synopsis of Clinical Dermatology*, 8th ed. New York, NY: McGraw Hill; 2017, Figure 2-17.)

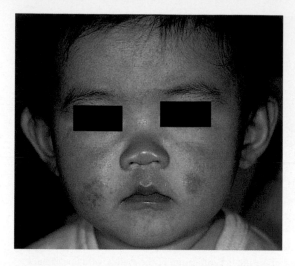

FIGURE 2-21. Bilateral red and orange papules and plaques on the cheeks of an Asian child, with mild pink erythema of the nasal tip and mid-upper cutaneous lip. (Reproduced with permission from Milgrom EC, Usatine RP, Tan RA, et al. *Practical Allergy.* Philadelphia, PA: Elsevier; 2004, Figure 3-5.)

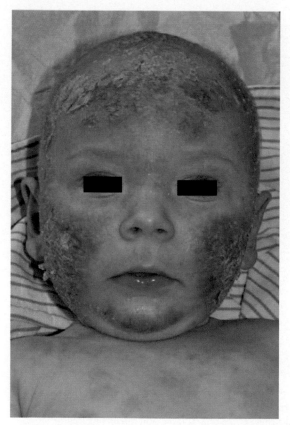

FIGURE 2-22. Crusted red patches and plaques with background erythema on the forehead, cheeks, and chin of a White baby. (Reproduced with permission from Fölster-Holst R, Wollenberg A: Atopic Dermatitis in Infants and Toddlers: A Diagnostic Challenge in Daily Practice. *Curr Derm Rep.* 2017;6:230–240.)

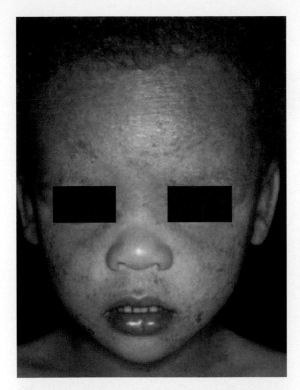

FIGURE 2-23. Pink and brown lichenified scaly patches and plaques on the face of a Hispanic child, with overlying scattered excoriations and notable sparing of the nose, medial cheeks, and chin. (From Taylor SC, Kelly AP, Lim HW, et al. *Taylor and Kelly's Dermatology for Skin of Color*, 2nd ed. New York, NY: McGraw Hill; 2016, Figure 95-6. Reproduced with permission from Dr. Tania Cestari.)

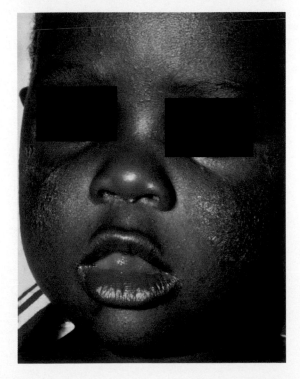

FIGURE 2-24. Deeply pigmented dark-brown scaly plaques with fine papules seen along the glabella and forehead of a Black infant, with notable sparing of the nose and medial cheeks. (From Taylor SC, Kelly AP, Lim HW, et al. *Taylor and Kelly's Dermatology for Skin of Color*, 2nd ed. New York, NY: McGraw Hill; 2016, Figure 95-4. Reproduced with permission from Barbara Leppard.)

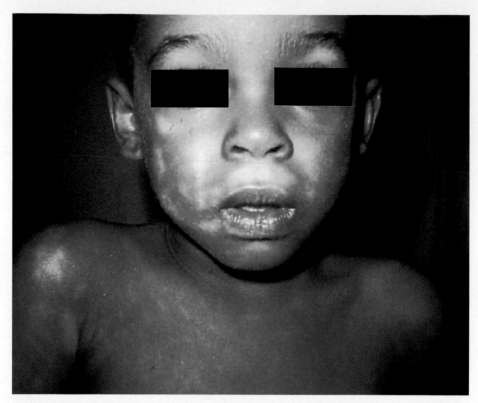

FIGURE 2-25. Ill-defined hypopigmented patches on the cheeks and upper lip, with a few fine papules overlying the glabella. The pigmentary changes are consistent with postinflammatory pigmentation that can occur with atopic dermatitis in a person with darker skin. (Reproduced with permission from Prose NS, Kristal L. *Weinberg's Color Atlas of Pediatric Dermatology*, 5th ed. New York, NY: McGraw Hill; 2017, Figure 27-20.)

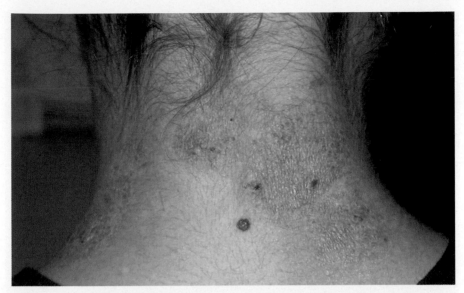

FIGURE 2-26. Nummular, pink, scaly lichenified plaques with peripheral violaceous hue on the posterior neck, with overlying scattered excoriations in a person with lighter skin of color. (Reproduced with permission from Milgrom EC, Usatine RP, Tan RA, et al. *Practical Allergy*. Philadelphia, PA: Elsevier; 2004, Figure 3-29.)

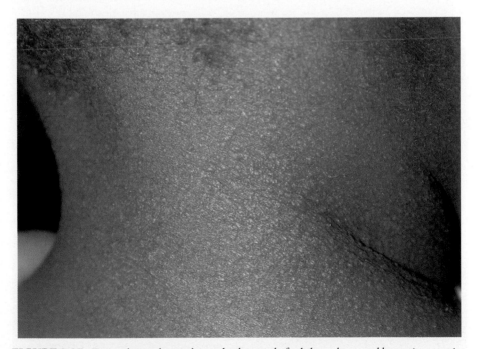

FIGURE 2-27. Fine scaly papules overlying a background of subtle erythema and hyperpigmentation on the posterior and lateral neck. (From Usatine RP, Smith MA, Mayeaux EJ Jr, et al. *The Color Atlas and Synopsis of Family Medicine*, 3rd ed. New York, NY: McGraw Hill; 2019, Figure 151-6. Reproduced with permission from Richard P. Usatine, MD.)

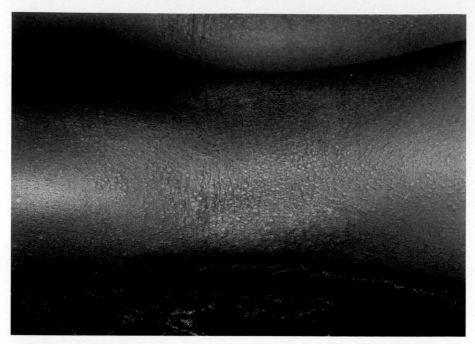

FIGURE 2-28. Fine skin-colored and dark-brown–gray papules overlying a background of hyperpigmentation and lichenification. (Reproduced with permission from Wolff K, Johnson RA, Saavedra AP, et al. *Fitzpatrick's Color Atlas and Synopsis of Clinical Dermatology*, 8th ed. New York, NY: McGraw Hill; 2017, Figure 2-14B.)

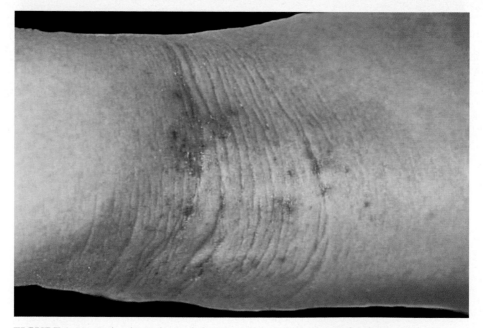

FIGURE 2-29. Red scaly patches and plaques overlying a background of pink lichenification. (Reproduced with permission from Wolff K, Johnson RA, Saavedra AP, et al. *Fitzpatrick's Color Atlas and Synopsis of Clinical Dermatology*, 8th ed. New York, NY: McGraw Hill; 2017, Figure 2-14A.)

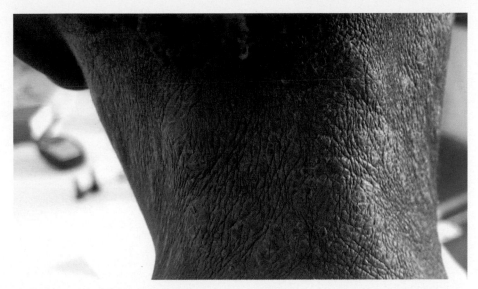

FIGURE 2-30. Diffuse dark-brown thickened velvety plaques on the posterior neck signifying chronic changes of atopic dermatitis. (Reproduced with permission from Taylor SC, Kelly AP, Lim HW, et al. *Taylor and Kelly's Dermatology for Skin of Color*, 2nd ed. New York, NY: McGraw Hill; 2016, Figure 86-14.)

KEY POINTS

- Psoriatic morphologies can include plaque, inverse, pustular, guttate, and erythrodermic psoriasis.

- Variants of active psoriasis can differ in color and thickness of scale across different racial/ethnic groups.

- In lighter skin, active disease is typically pink and red in contrast to being violaceous and brown in darker skin.

- Chronic treated psoriasis can result in dyspigmentation more commonly seen in skin of color, which can span the spectrum from postinflammatory hyperpigmentation to hypopigmentation.

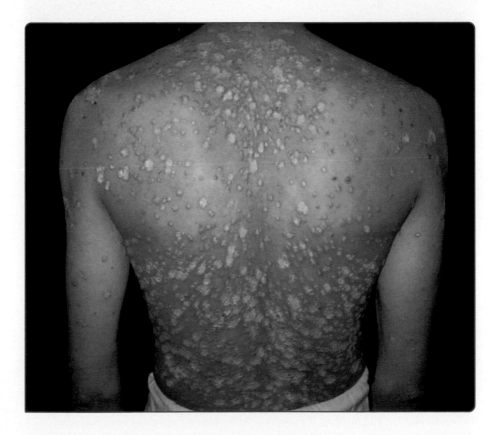

Scalp Psoriasis

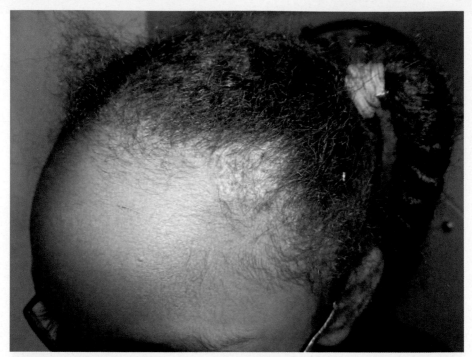

FIGURE 3-1. Well-demarcated, annular gray plaque along the left hairline, with overlying scale and lacking visible erythema. (Reproduced with permission from Taylor SC, Kelly AP, Lim HW, et al. *Taylor and Kelly's Dermatology for Skin of Color*, 2nd ed. New York, NY: McGraw Hill; 2016, Figure 84-1.)

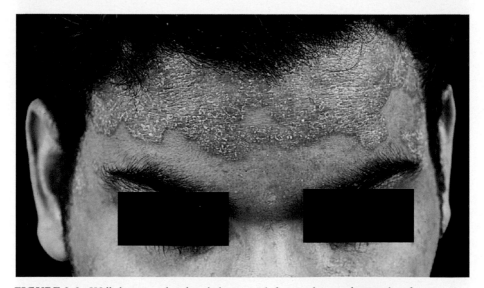

FIGURE 3-2. Well-demarcated pink-red plaques with fine overlying scale extending from the hairline onto the mid-forehead, also involving the temples, eyebrows, and periorbital skin. (Reproduced with permission from Wolff K, Johnson RA, Saavedra AP, et al. *Fitzpatrick's Color Atlas and Synopsis of Clinical Dermatology*, 8th ed. New York, NY: McGraw Hill; 2017, Figure 3-8.)

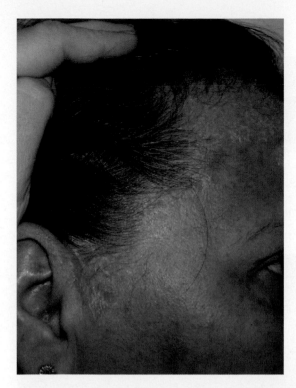

FIGURE 3-3. Light-pink confluent plaques with fine overlying white scale extending from the preauricular scalp along the frontal hairline and forehead. Along the perimeter of the plaque, a few macules of hyperpigmentation and hypopigmentation are also visible. (From Taylor SC, Kelly AP, Lim HW, et al. *Taylor and Kelly's Dermatology for Skin of Color*, 2nd ed. New York, NY: McGraw Hill; 2016, Figure 95-48. Reproduced with permission from Barbara Leppard.)

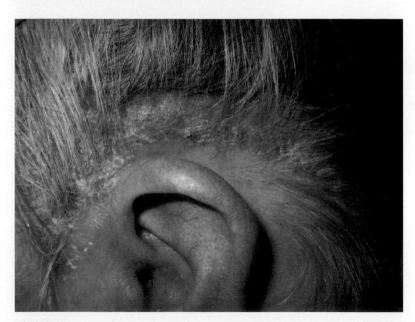

FIGURE 3-4. Confluent pink-red plaques with overlying white scale extending along the hairline, starting at the preauricular scalp. (Reproduced with permission from Soutor C, Hordinsky MK. *Clinical Dermatology*. New York, NY: McGraw Hill; 2013, Figure 9-3.)

Plaque Psoriasis

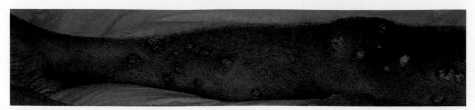

FIGURE 3-5. Violaceous and dark-brown–gray guttate papules and plaques with overlying white scale along the anterior lower extremities, resembling a hypertrophic lichen planus-like presentation. (Reproduced with permission from Taylor SC, Kelly AP, Lim HW, et al. *Taylor and Kelly's Dermatology for Skin of Color*, 2nd ed. New York, NY: McGraw Hill; 2016, Figure 24-13.)

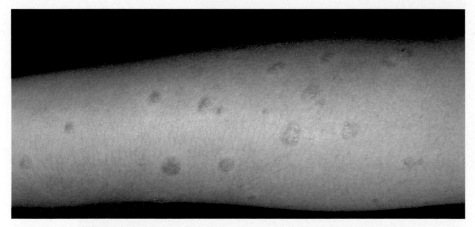

FIGURE 3-6. Well-demarcated light-pink guttate plaques with minimal visible overlying scale on an upper extremity. A few of the plaques are surrounded by a halo of hypopigmented skin. (From Usatine RP, Smith MA, Mayeaux EJ Jr, et al. *The Color Atlas and Synopsis of Family Medicine*, 3rd ed. New York, NY: McGraw Hill; 2019, Figure 158-5A. Reproduced with permission from Richard P. Usatine, MD.)

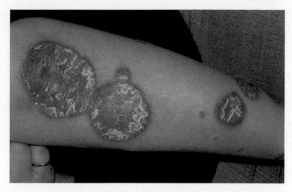

FIGURE 3-7. Well-demarcated bright-pink annular plaques with overlying micaceous scale on the extensor upper extremity. (From Usatine RP, Smith MA, Mayeaux EJ Jr, et al. *The Color Atlas and Synopsis of Family Medicine*, 3rd ed. New York, NY: McGraw Hill; 2019, Figure 158-1. Reproduced with permission from Richard P. Usatine, MD.)

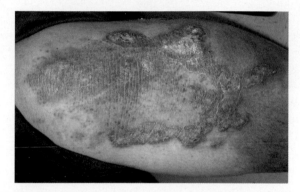

FIGURE 3-8. Hispanic man with violaceous to gray-brown hyperkeratotic plaques and background lichenified pink-purple skin changes extending from the knee down to the anterior shin. (From Usatine RP, Smith MA, Mayeaux EJ Jr, et al. *The Color Atlas and Synopsis of Family Medicine*, 3rd ed. New York, NY: McGraw Hill; 2019, Figure 158-13. Reproduced with permission from Richard P. Usatine, MD.)

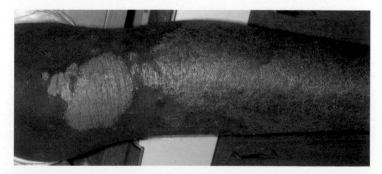

FIGURE 3-9. Silvery-white scaly plaques, which are well demarcated on the knee and confluent along the anterior shin where diffuse background violaceous discoloration is also notable. (From Usatine RP, Smith MA, Mayeaux EJ Jr, et al. *The Color Atlas and Synopsis of Family Medicine*, 3rd ed. New York, NY: McGraw Hill; 2019, Figure 158-12. Reproduced with permission from Richard P. Usatine, MD.)

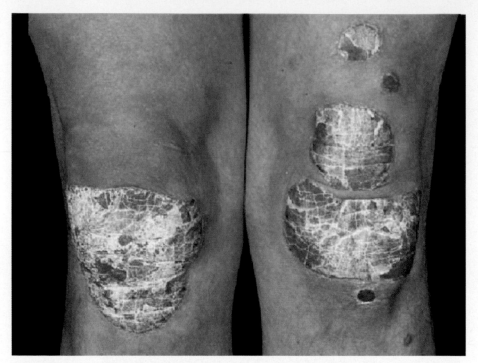

FIGURE 3-10. Well-demarcated pink plaques with overlying hyperkeratotic scale. Note the lack of lichenification and surrounding discoloration. (Reproduced with permission from Wolff K. *Fitzpatrick's Color Atlas and Synopsis of Clinical Dermatology*, 5th ed. New York, NY: McGraw Hill; 1999, Figure 43-1B.)

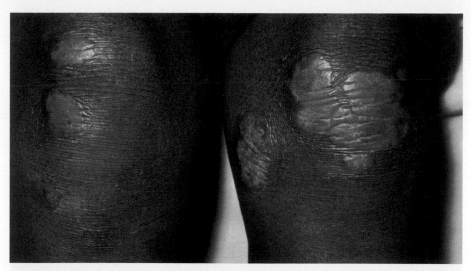

FIGURE 3-11. Well-demarcated pink plaques with areas of overlying brown pigmentation lacking overlying scale and with background lichenification in a person with darker skin. (From Taylor SC, Kelly AP, Lim HW, et al. *Taylor and Kelly's Dermatology for Skin of Color*, 2nd ed. New York, NY: McGraw Hill; 2016, Figure 95-46. Reproduced with permission from Barbara Leppard.)

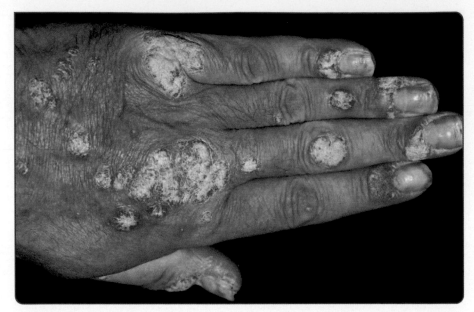

FIGURE 3-12. Dorsal hand with numerous discrete hyperkeratotic pink plaques along the dorsal hand and digits. Note the plaques extending along the proximal and lateral nail folds as well as the onycholysis and oil spots of the left thumbnail. (From Kang S, Amagai M, Bruckner AL, et al. *Fitzpatrick's Dermatology*, 9th ed. New York, NY: McGraw Hill; 2019, Figure 28-1D. Reproduced with permission from Dr. Johann Gudjonsson and Mr. Harrold Carter.)

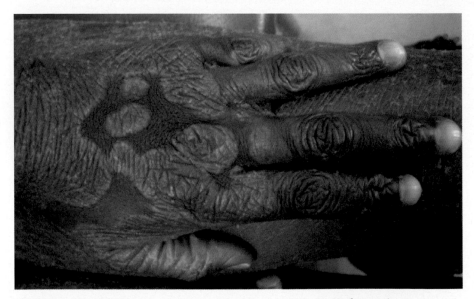

FIGURE 3-13. Well-demarcated plaques with variegated colors ranging from violaceous to pink-brown and fine overlying scale on the dorsal hand and digits. On the third dorsal digit is a hypopigmented patch signifying postinflammatory hypopigmentation. (Reproduced with permission from Prose NS, Kristal L. *Weinberg's Color Atlas of Pediatric Dermatology*, 5th ed. New York, NY: McGraw Hill; 2017, Figure 18-12.)

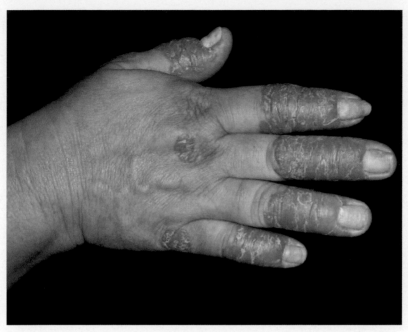

FIGURE 3-14. Well-demarcated bright-pink plaques with micaceous scale extending from the proximal interphalangeal joints to the distal fingertips as well as on the metacarpophalangeal joints. Note the pitting and oil spots visible on the fingernails. (From Usatine RP, Smith MA, Mayeaux EJ Jr, et al. *The Color Atlas and Synopsis of Family Medicine*, 3rd ed. New York, NY: McGraw Hill; 2019, Figure 158-28. Reproduced with permission from Richard P. Usatine, MD.)

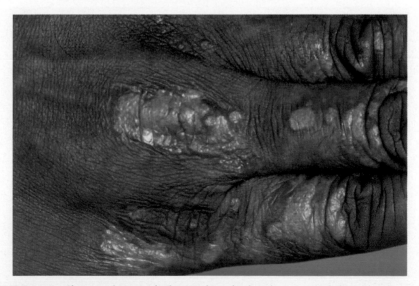

FIGURE 3-15. Chronic salmon-pink plaques along the dorsal metacarpophalangeal and extending to the proximal interphalangeal joints, with surrounding hypopigmented and hyperpigmented patches. Note the paucity of scale, which may signify partially treated chronic disease. (From Taylor SC, Kelly AP, Lim HW, et al. *Taylor and Kelly's Dermatology for Skin of Color*, 2nd ed. New York, NY: McGraw Hill; 2016, Figure 24-2. Reproduced with permission from the National Skin Centre, Singapore.)

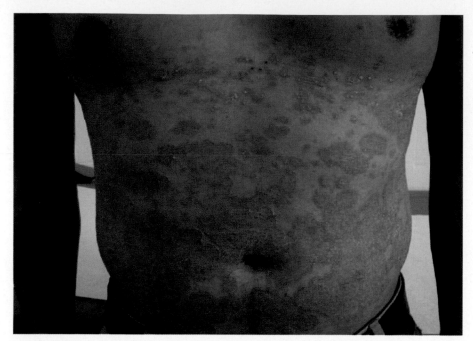

FIGURE 3-16. Trunk with large confluent bright-pink plaques with a brown rim. (Reproduced with permission from Kang S, Amagai M, Bruckner AL, et al. *Fitzpatrick's Dermatology*, 9th ed. New York, NY: McGraw Hill; 2019, Figure 1-4.)

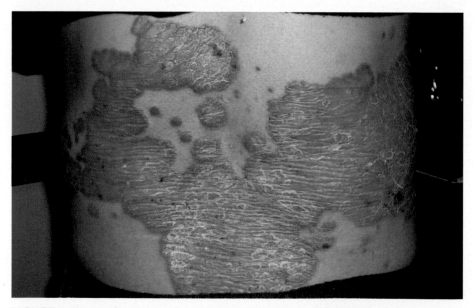

FIGURE 3-17. Trunk with large discrete bright-pink plaques with a violaceous rim and overlying scale and scattered excoriations. (From Usatine RP, Smith MA, Mayeaux EJ Jr, et al. *The Color Atlas and Synopsis of Family Medicine*, 3rd ed. New York, NY: McGraw Hill; 2019, Figure 158-3. Reproduced with permission from Richard P. Usatine, MD.)

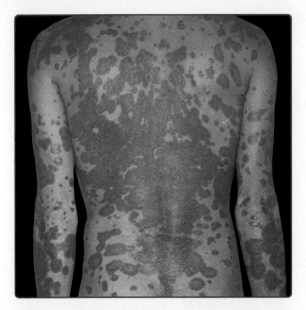

FIGURE 3-18. Posterior trunk with bright-pink–red confluent plaques. (From Kang S, Amagai M, Bruckner AL, et al. *Fitzpatrick's Dermatology*, 9th ed. New York, NY: McGraw Hill; 2019, Figure 199-2A. Reproduced with permission from Wolff K, Hönigsmann H, Gschnait F, et al. Photochemotherapy of psoriasis: clinical experiences with 152 patients. *Dtsch Med Wochenschr*. 1975;100(48):2471-2477.)

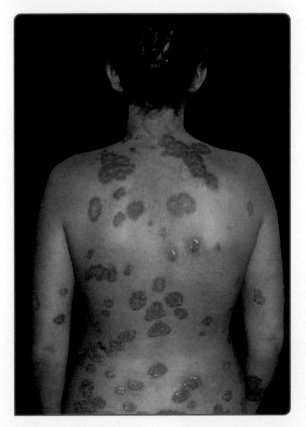

FIGURE 3-19. Posterior trunk with fiery red discrete scaly plaques, which are more confluent on the upper mid-back. (From Kang S, Amagai M, Bruckner AL, et al. *Fitzpatrick's Dermatology*, 9th ed. New York, NY: McGraw Hill; 2019, Figure 28-1A. Reproduced with permission from Dr. Johann Gudjonsson and Mr. Harrold Carter.)

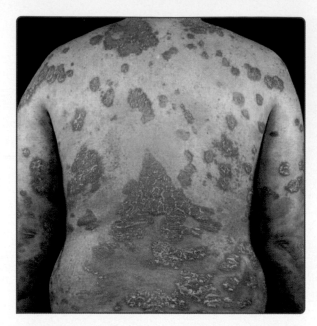

FIGURE 3-20. Posterior trunk and upper extremity with large confluent pink-brown scaly plaques, which vary in size and shape. (From Kang S, Amagai M, Bruckner AL, et al. *Fitzpatrick's Dermatology*, 9th ed. New York, NY: McGraw Hill; 2019, Figure 28-1C. Reproduced with permission from Dr. Johann Gudjonsson and Mr. Harrold Carter.)

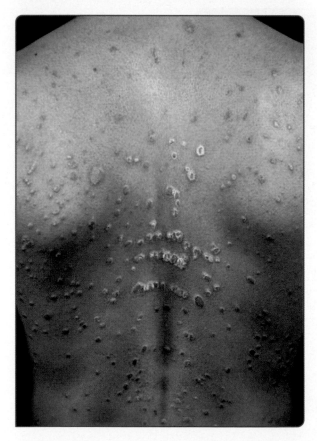

FIGURE 3-21. Posterior trunk with discrete guttate violaceous scaly plaques with lichen planus-like presentation. (From Kang S, Amagai M, Bruckner AL, et al. *Fitzpatrick's Dermatology*, 9th ed. New York, NY: McGraw Hill; 2019, Figure 28-5C. Reproduced with permission from Drs. Johann Gudjonsson and Trilokraj Tejasvi, Mr. Harrold Carter, and Ms. Laura Vangoor.)

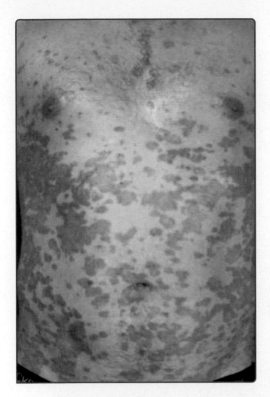

FIGURE 3-22. Pink-salmon–colored plaques scattered diffusely on the anterior trunk. (From Kang S, Amagai M, Bruckner AL, et al. *Fitzpatrick's Dermatology*, 9th ed. New York, NY: McGraw Hill; 2019, Figure 198-3A. Reproduced with permission from Herbert Hönigsmann, MD.)

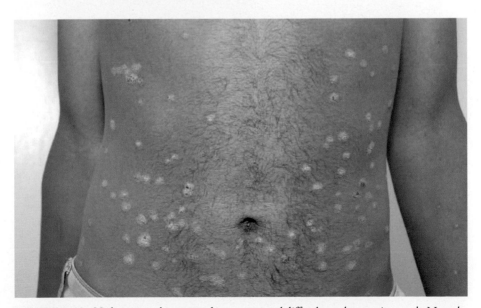

FIGURE 3-23. Violaceous scaly guttate plaques scattered diffusely on the anterior trunk. Note the excoriations visible on several of the plaques. (From Usatine RP, Smith MA, Mayeaux EJ Jr, et al. *The Color Atlas and Synopsis of Family Medicine*, 3rd ed. New York, NY: McGraw Hill; 2019, Figure 158-20. Reproduced with permission from Richard P. Usatine, MD.)

Pustular psoriasis

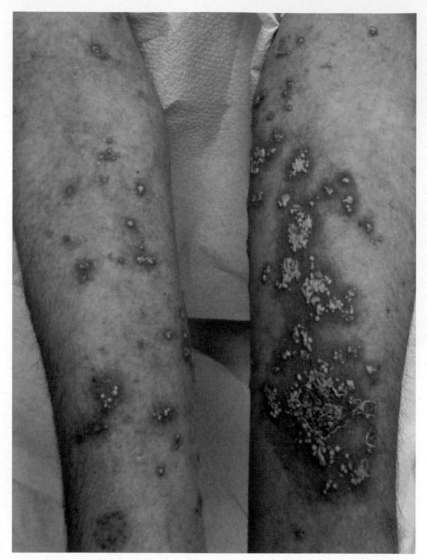

FIGURE 3-24. Bright-pink to red macules and patches with overlying scale and yellow pustules, some of which are clustered along the bilateral ventral forearms. (From Usatine RP, Smith MA, Mayeaux EJ Jr, et al. *The Color Atlas and Synopsis of Family Medicine*, 3rd ed. New York, NY: McGraw Hill; 2019, Figure 158-31A. Reproduced with permission from Robert T. Gilson, MD.)

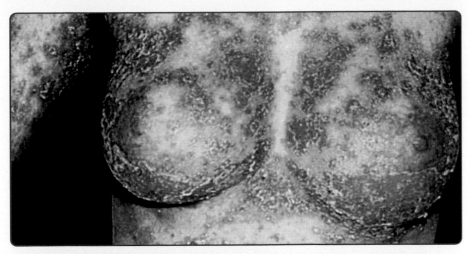

FIGURE 3-25. Crusted pustules and plaques with a background erythema in a person of color. (From Kang S, Amagai M, Bruckner AL, et al. *Fitzpatrick's Dermatology*, 9th ed. New York, NY: McGraw Hill; 2019, Figure 199-4. Reproduced with permission from Hönigsmann H, Gschnait F, Konrad K, Wolff K. Photochemotherapy for pustular psoriasis (von Zumbusch). *Br J Dermatol*. 1977;97(2):119-126.)

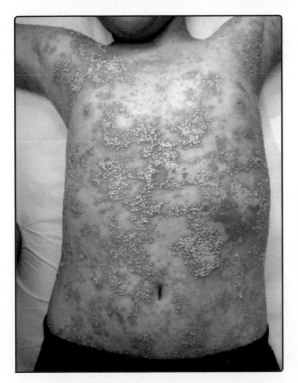

FIGURE 3-26. Anterior trunk with scattered large, confluent, pink-salmon–colored patches with overlying clustered pustules. (From Kang S, Amagai M, Bruckner AL, et al. *Fitzpatrick's Dermatology*, 9th ed. New York, NY: McGraw Hill; 2019, Figure 39-5A. Reproduced with permission from Eskin-Schwartz M, Basel-Vanagaite L, David M, et al. Intrafamilial variation in clinical phenotype of CARD14-related psoriasis. *Acta Derm Venereol*. 2016;96(7):885-887.)

Inverse Psoriasis

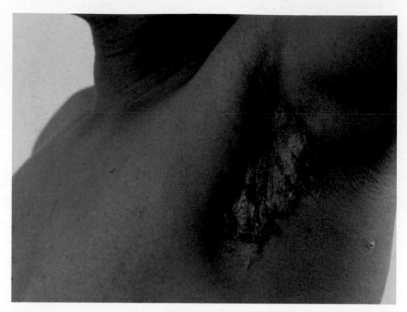

FIGURE 3-27. Left axilla and inframammary skin with confluent violaceous and dark-brown plaques with diffuse overlying scale. (Reproduced with permission from Taylor SC, Kelly AP, Lim HW, et al. *Taylor and Kelly's Dermatology for Skin of Color*, 2nd ed. New York, NY: McGraw Hill; 2016, Figure 24-9.)

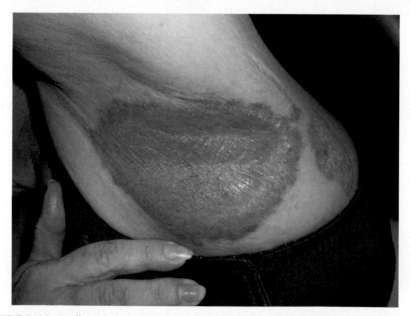

FIGURE 3-28. Axilla with discrete bright-pink plaque with peripheral scale. (From Usatine RP, Smith MA, Mayeaux EJ Jr, et al. *The Color Atlas and Synopsis of Family Medicine*, 3rd ed. New York, NY: McGraw Hill; 2019, Figure 158-6. Reproduced with permission from Richard P. Usatine, MD.)

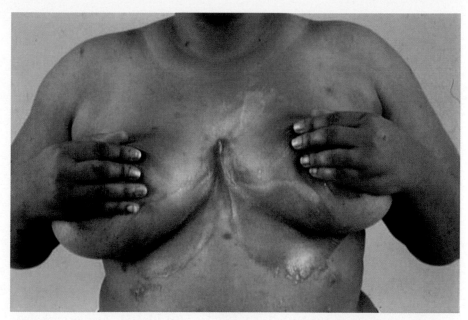

FIGURE 3-29. Inferior breasts and inframammary skin with large, discrete, smooth, confluent violaceous patches lacking overlying scale. (Reproduced with permission from Taylor SC, Kelly AP, Lim HW, et al. *Taylor and Kelly's Dermatology for Skin of Color*, 2nd ed. New York, NY: McGraw Hill; 2016, Figure 24-8.)

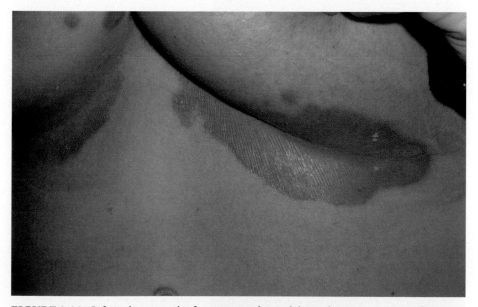

FIGURE 3-30. Inferior breasts and inframammary skin with large, discrete, smooth, confluent pink patches with brown rim and lacking overlying scale. (From Usatine RP, Smith MA, Mayeaux EJ Jr, et al. *The Color Atlas and Synopsis of Family Medicine*, 3rd ed. New York, NY: McGraw Hill; 2019, Figure 158-2. Reproduced with permission from Richard P. Usatine, MD.)

Additional Presentations of Psoriasis

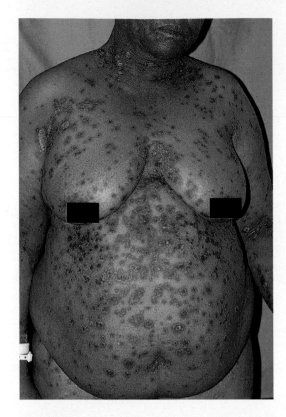

FIGURE 3-31. Anterior trunk of a pregnant woman with diffuse scattered violaceous and red-brown patches and plaques, many of which have central crusting and scale. (Reproduced with permission from Burgin S. *Guidebook to Dermatologic Diagnosis*. New York, NY: McGraw Hill; 2021, Figure 2-36.)

Erythrodermic Psoriasis

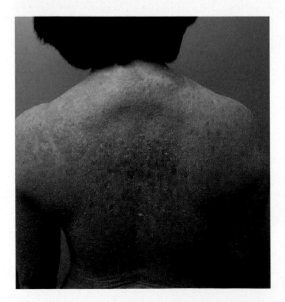

FIGURE 3-32. Diffuse pink scaly patches covering the back and posterior upper extremities with few areas of sparing in an Asian woman. (Reproduced with permission from Jackson-Richards D, Pandya AG. *Dermatology Atlas for Skin of Color*. Berlin Heidelberg: Springer-Verlag; 2014.)

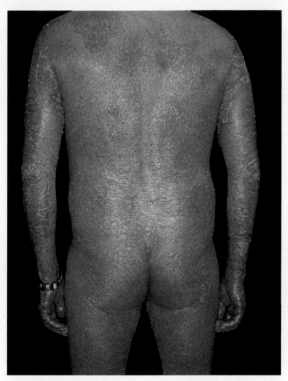

FIGURE 3-33. Diffuse pink-red lichenified patch covering posterior trunk and upper extremity with overlying white scale and desquamation with sparing of only the upper back. (From Usatine RP, Smith MA, Mayeaux EJ Jr, et al. *The Color Atlas and Synopsis of Family Medicine*, 3rd ed. New York, NY: McGraw Hill; 2019, Figure 158-8. Reproduced with permission from Richard P. Usatine, MD.)

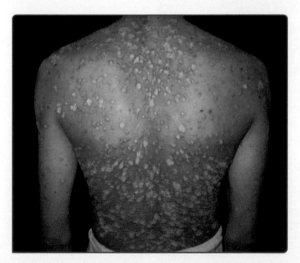

FIGURE 3-34. Posterior trunk with guttate light pink scaly plaques and a violaceous rim, which are more confluent on the lower back and in a pityriasis rosea-like distribution. (From Kang S, Amagai M, Bruckner AL, et al. *Fitzpatrick's Dermatology*, 9th ed. New York, NY: McGraw Hill; 2019, Figure 28-5D. Reproduced with permission from Drs. Johann Gudjonsson and Trilokraj Tejasvi, Mr. Harrold Carter, and Ms. Laura Vangoor.)

Postinflammatory Pigment Alteration from Psoriasis

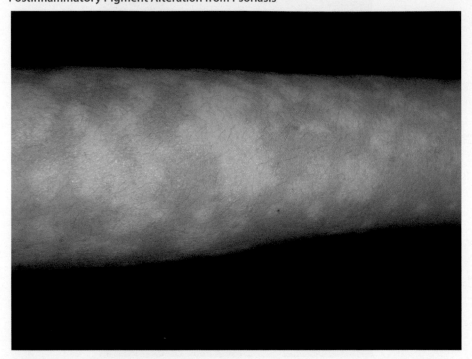

FIGURE 3-35. Hypopigmented macules and patches with background pink areas indicative of active psoriatic disease seen along an extremity. (From Usatine RP, Smith MA, Mayeaux EJ Jr, et al. *The Color Atlas and Synopsis of Family Medicine*, 3rd ed. New York, NY: McGraw Hill; 2019, Figure 110-21. Reproduced with permission from Richard P. Usatine, MD.)

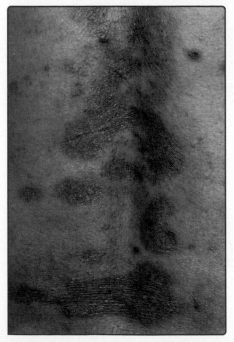

FIGURE 3-36. Posterior trunk with dark-brown patches representing postinflammatory change from resolving psoriasis. (Reproduced with permission from Kang S, Amagai M, Bruckner AL, et al. *Fitzpatrick's Dermatology*, 9th ed. New York, NY: McGraw Hill; 2019, Figure 77-21B.)

KEY POINTS

- Contact dermatitis can commonly occur in many body areas including periorally, periocularly, periumbilically, and on the extremities with morphology varying from vesicular and bullous to patches and even plaques in chronic disease.

- In lighter skin, active contact dermatitis is typically pink or red, while in darker skin, it can vary from magenta to violaceous and brown. Often, features of active and chronic disease can be seen simultaneously.

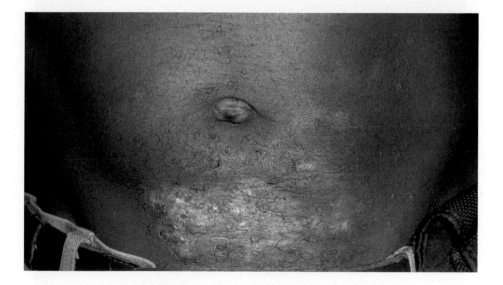

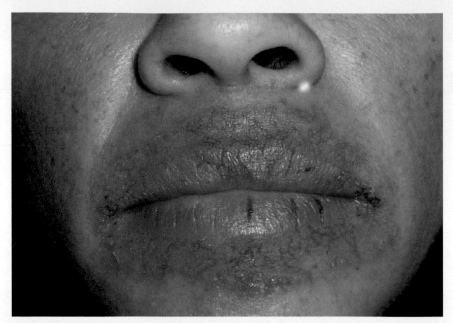

FIGURE 4-1. Perioral erythema with yellow crusting at the lateral commisures and under the mid-lower lip. Note several linear fissures on the mucosal lips. The patient had been using Carmex and licking her lips. (From Usatine RP, Smith MA, Mayeaux EJ Jr, et al. *The Color Atlas and Synopsis of Family Medicine*, 3rd ed. New York, NY: McGraw Hill; 2019, Figure 152-21. Reproduced with permission from Richard P. Usatine, MD.)

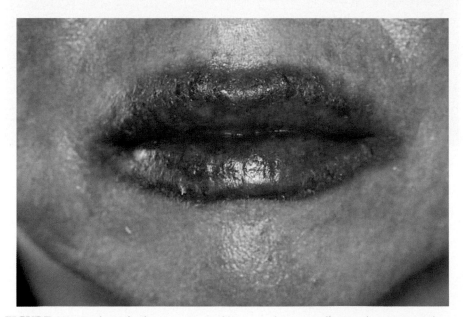

FIGURE 4-2. Bright-pink edematous mucosal lips extending periorally onto the cutaneous skin with scaling and crusting along the vermillion border. (Reproduced with permission from Wolff K, Johnson RA, Saavedra AP, et al. *Fitzpatrick's Color Atlas and Synopsis of Clinical Dermatology*, 8th ed. New York, NY: McGraw Hill; 2017, Figure 2-5.)

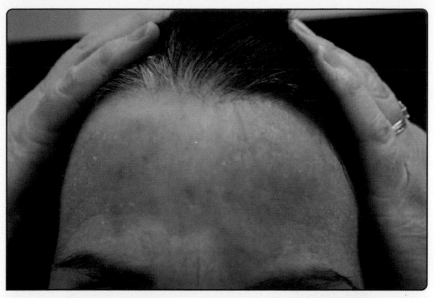

FIGURE 4-3. Light-pink to salmon-colored large, scaly, confluent patch along the forehead, with sparing along the hairline and above the eyebrows. This is secondary to para-pheylenediamine. (Reproduced with permission from Kang S, Amagai M, Bruckner AL, et al. *Fitzpatrick's Dermatology*, 9th ed. New York, NY: McGraw Hill; 2019, Figure 24-2B.)

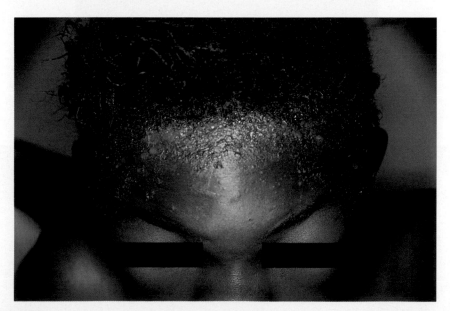

FIGURE 4-4. Dark-brown confluent vesicular plaque along the hairline and on the forehead, with areas of overlying pink macules and brown crusting. On the central forehead are several scattered skin-colored to brown pinpoint papules. Note the intensity of the black hair dye along the hairline. This is secondary to para-phenylenediamine. (Reproduced with permission from Taylor SC, Kelly AP, Lim HW, et al. *Taylor and Kelly's Dermatology for Skin of Color*, 2nd ed. New York, NY: McGraw Hill; 2016, Figure 28-4A.)

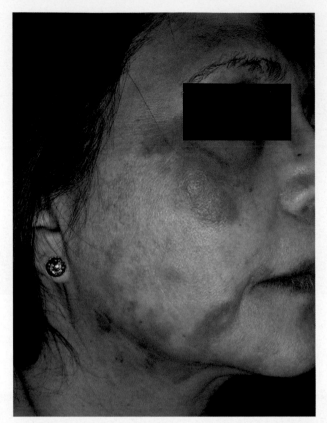

FIGURE 4-5. Numerous scattered patches and plaques on the right cheek and jawline, ranging from fuchsia on the malar prominence to dusky pink along the jawline and neck in a person with lighter skin of color. This is secondary to contact dermatitis from Balsam of Peru and formaldehyde. (From Usatine RP, Smith MA, Mayeaux EJ Jr, et al. *The Color Atlas and Synopsis of Family Medicine*, 3rd ed. New York, NY: McGraw Hill; 2019, Figure 152-19A. Reproduced with permission from Richard P. Usatine, MD.)

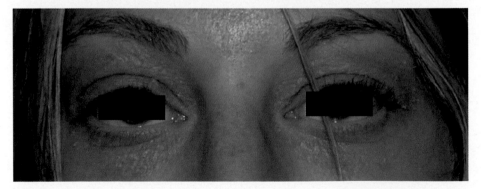

FIGURE 4-6. Bilateral periorbital edema with overlying pink- to salmon-colored lichenified scaly patches. This was secondary to fragrance. (Reproduced with permission from Baumann L, Saghari S, Weisberg E. *Cosmetic Dermatology: Principles and Practice*, 2nd ed. New York, NY: McGraw Hill; 2009, Figure 18-3.)

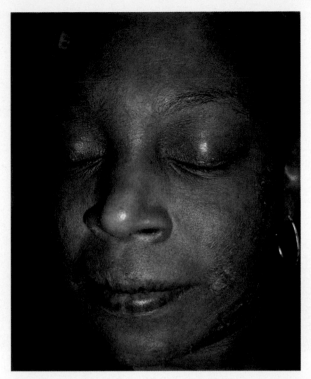

FIGURE 4-7. Pink-brown patches on the malar cheek with brown scaly plaques peripherally along the lateral aspect of the face in a person with darker skin of color. Note the background erythema on the cheek. This is secondary to Balsam of Peru and isothiazolinone in a young woman applying new moisturizer to the face. (From Usatine RP, Smith MA, Mayeaux EJ Jr, et al. *The Color Atlas and Synopsis of Family Medicine*, 3rd ed. New York, NY: McGraw Hill; 2019, Figure 152-19B. Reproduced with permission from Richard P. Usatine, MD.)

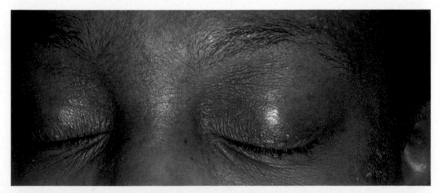

FIGURE 4-8. Pink to violaceous lichenified patches on the upper and lower eyelids with linear pink to purple pigmentation along the eyelid margins. Note the central area of sparing on both eyelids. This was secondary to Balsam of Peru and isothiazolinone in a young woman applying new moisturizer to the face. (From Usatine RP, Smith MA, Mayeaux EJ Jr, et al. *The Color Atlas and Synopsis of Family Medicine*, 3rd ed. New York, NY: McGraw Hill; 2019, Figure 152-19B. Reproduced with permission from Richard P. Usatine, MD.)

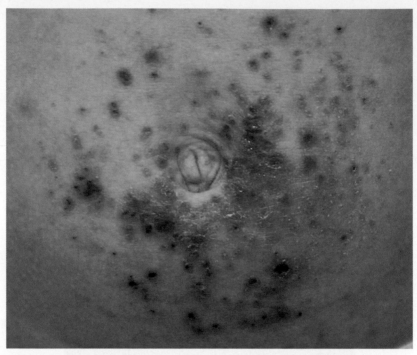

FIGURE 4-9. Periumbilical pink papules and plaques with overlying scaling and hemorrhagic crusting. This is secondary to nickel. (Reproduced with permission from Prose NS, Kristal L. *Weinberg's Color Atlas of Pediatric Dermatology*, 5th ed. New York, NY: McGraw Hill; 2017, Figure 10-12.)

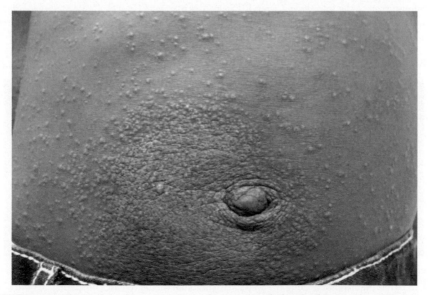

FIGURE 4-10. Periumbilical brown-pink, confluent, lichenified scaly plaque with peripheral scattered monomorphic papules on the abdomen. These changes can be seen acutely in response to nickel exposure. (Reproduced with permission from Soutor C, Hordinsky MK. *Clinical Dermatology.* New York, NY: McGraw Hill; 2013, Figure 2-2.)

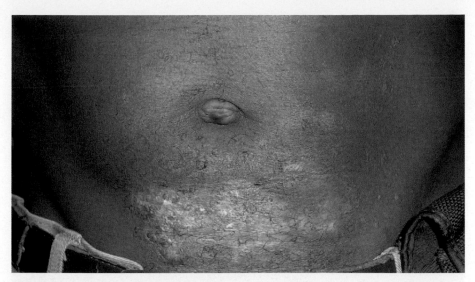

FIGURE 4-11. Infraumbilical pink-gray lichenified plaque with several peripheral brown-gray scaly macules consistent with chronic changes secondary to nickel. (From Usatine RP, Smith MA, Mayeaux EJ Jr, et al. *The Color Atlas and Synopsis of Family Medicine*, 3rd ed. New York, NY: McGraw Hill; 2019, Figure 152-5. Reproduced with permission from Richard P. Usatine, MD.)

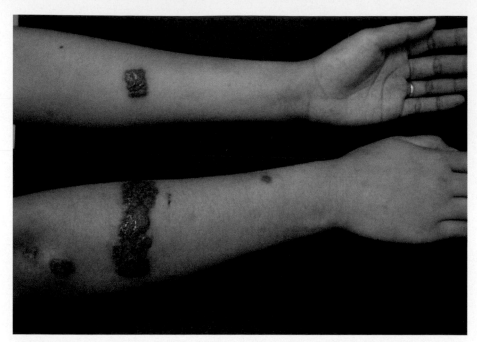

FIGURE 4-12. Violaceous well-demarcated edematous plaques on the bilateral forearms secondary to henna tattoo. (From Taylor SC, Kelly AP, Lim HW, et al. *Taylor and Kelly's Dermatology for Skin of Color*, 2nd ed. New York, NY: McGraw Hill; 2016, Figure 90-1. Reproduced with permission from Research Institute for Tropical Medicine, Department of Dermatology.)

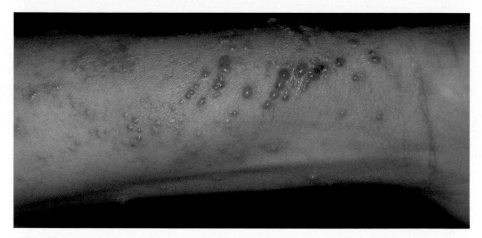

FIGURE 4-13. Numerous pink vesicles and papules in a linear morphology overlying a background of erythema. Superiorly several of the vesicles exhibit oozing of yellow serosanguinous fluid as well as yellow crusting. This represents an acute reaction to poison ivy. (From Usatine RP, Smith MA, Mayeaux EJ Jr, et al. *The Color Atlas and Synopsis of Family Medicine*, 3rd ed. New York, NY: McGraw Hill; 2019, Figure 152-16. Reproduced with permission from Richard P. Usatine, MD.)

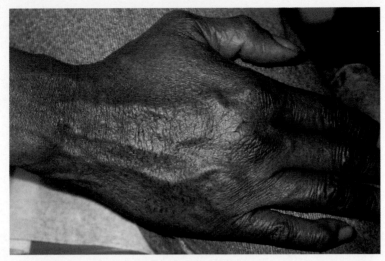

FIGURE 4-14. Pink-brown ill-defined lichenified plaque with overlying superficial linear fissures on the dorsal hand secondary to perfume. (From Usatine RP, Smith MA, Mayeaux EJ Jr, Chumley HS. *The Color Atlas and Synopsis of Family Medicine*, 3rd ed. New York, NY: McGraw Hill; 2019, Figure 153-2. Reproduced with permission from Richard P. Usatine, MD.)

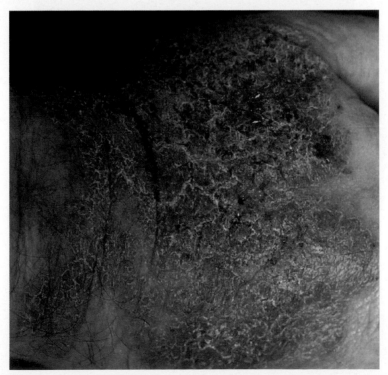

FIGURE 4-15. Pink and red lichenified scaly plaques with several superficial erosions and fissures on the dorsal hand of a construction worker secondary to a chromate allergy. (Reproduced with permission from Wolff K, Johnson RA, Saavedra AP, et al. *Fitzpatrick's Color Atlas and Synopsis of Clinical Dermatology*, 8th ed. New York, NY: McGraw Hill; 2017, Figure 2-6.)

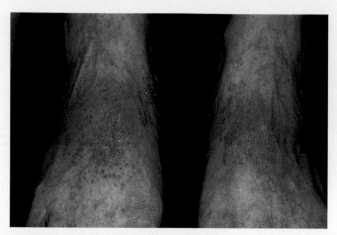

FIGURE 4-16. Red papules and vesicles overlying a background of erythema along the bilateral dorsal feet secondary to allergic contact dermatitis from new shoes. (From Usatine RP, Smith MA, Mayeaux EJ Jr, et al. *The Color Atlas and Synopsis of Family Medicine*, 3rd ed. New York, NY: McGraw Hill; 2019, Figure 152-11. Reproduced with permission from Milgrom EC, Usatine RP, Tan RA, et al. *Practical Allergy*. Philadelphia, PA: Elsevier; 2004, Figure 4-22.)

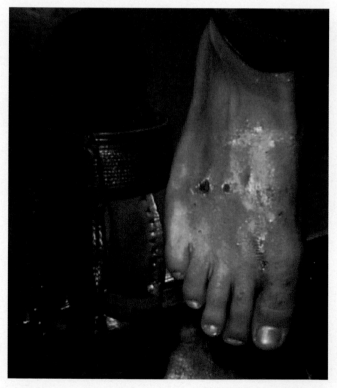

FIGURE 4-17. Red erosions and patches along the dorsal foot and great dorsal toe aligning with the areas of contact from a sandal. This is secondary to the tanning agent/dye in the sandal. (Reproduced with permission from Prose NS, Kristal L. *Weinberg's Color Atlas of Pediatric Dermatology*, 5th ed. New York, NY: McGraw Hill; 2017, Figure 10-9.)

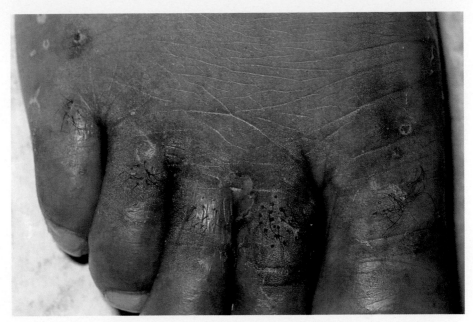

FIGURE 4-18. Dark-brown ill-defined patches along the dorsal toes and superior dorsal foot. (Reproduced with permission from Taylor SC, Kelly AP, Lim HW, et al. *Taylor and Kelly's Dermatology for Skin of Color*, 2nd ed. New York, NY: McGraw Hill; 2016, Figure 28-3.)

KEY POINTS

- Pityriasis lichenoides chronica (PLC) is a lymphoproliferative papulosquamous condition with varying presentations.

- In lighter skin, it tends to present with pink to red papules and macules with background erythema and variable scale.

- In darker skin, presentation also includes scaly papules and macules but varies in color from violaceous and dark brown to hypopigmented. This often resolves with postinflammatory pigment alteration.

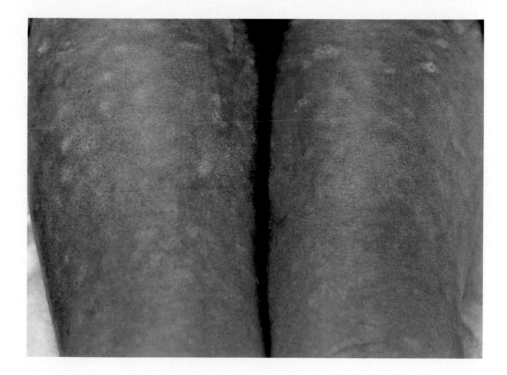

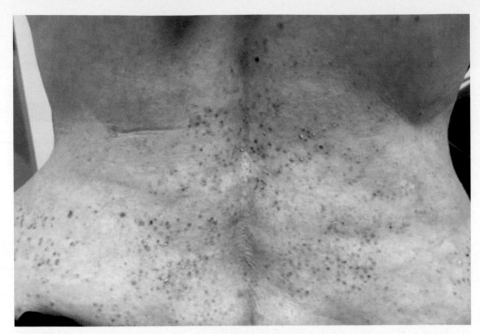

FIGURE 5-1. Fuschia-pink papules scattered on the mid to lower back, lacking scale and with significant background erythema. (From Usatine RP, Smith MA, Mayeaux EJ Jr, et al. *The Color Atlas and Synopsis of Family Medicine*, 3rd ed. New York, NY: McGraw Hill; 2019, Figure 194-9. Reproduced with permission from Richard P. Usatine, MD.)

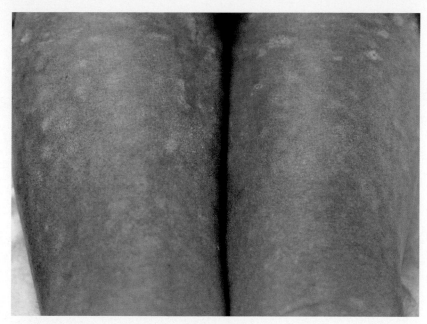

FIGURE 5-2. Anterior thighs showing diffuse hyperpigmented and hypopigmented patches with overlying scale and background erythema. (Reproduced with permission from Prose NS, Kristal L. *Weinberg's Color Atlas of Pediatric Dermatology*, 5th ed. New York, NY: McGraw Hill; 2017, Figure 12-43.)

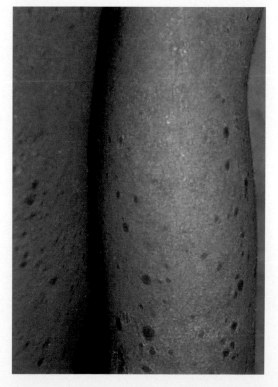

FIGURE 5-3. Purple-brown papules and macules with diffuse overlying and background scale. (Reproduced with permission from Burgin S. *Guidebook to Dermatologic Diagnosis*. New York, NY: McGraw Hill; 2021, Figure 4-11C.)

KEY POINTS

- Pityriasis rosea can present with various morphologies and includes numerous variants.

- In darker skin, this can be papulosquamous and pink to brown, violaceous, or gray in color, in contrast to lighter skin, where it is typically pink to salmon colored.

- In darker skin, there is also a papular morphology variant that can be seen.

- The herald patch in darker skin often has a darker central hue, which can range from violaceous to brown to gray with a lighter peripheral rim. The overlying scale can also be more difficult to appreciate in darker skin.

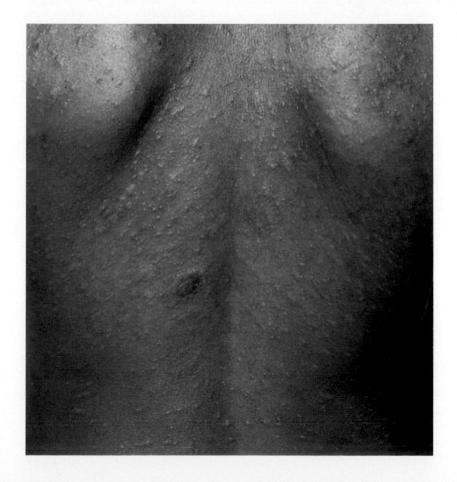

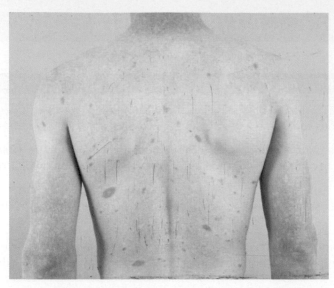

FIGURE 6-1. Discrete pink papules and plaques in a Christmas-tree distribution on the back, representing classic presentation of pityriasis rosea in a lighter-skinned person. (Reproduced with permission from Taylor SC, Kelly AP, Lim HW, et al. *Taylor and Kelly's Dermatology for Skin of Color*, 2nd ed. New York, NY: McGraw Hill; 2016, Figure 25-4B.)

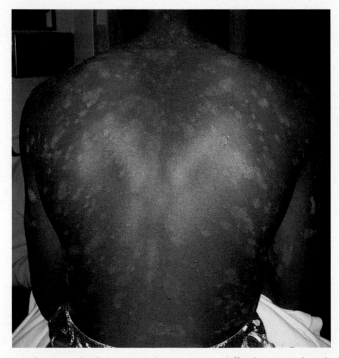

FIGURE 6-2. Pink-gray scaly plaques mimicking psoriasis, diffusely scattered on the back and posterior upper extremities. (From Usatine RP, Smith MA, Mayeaux EJ Jr, et al. *The Color Atlas and Synopsis of Family Medicine*, 3rd ed. New York, NY: McGraw Hill; 2019, Figure 159-7. Reproduced with permission from E.J. Mayeaux, Jr., MD.)

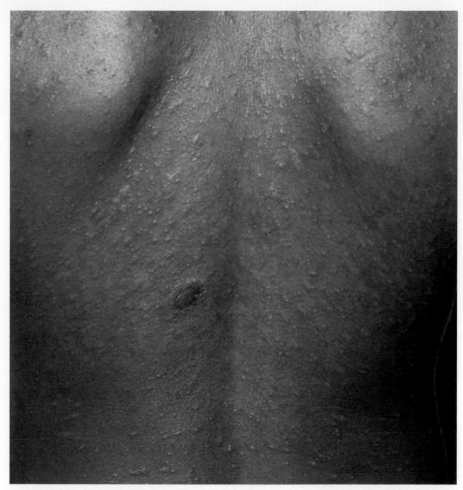

FIGURE 6-3. Pink papules in a Christmas-tree distribution along Langer lines, with a prominent red-brown plaque on the left mid-back representing the herald patch. (Reproduced with permission from Kang S, Amagai M, Bruckner AL, et al. *Fitzpatrick's Dermatology*, 9th ed. New York, NY: McGraw Hill; 2019, Figure 31-8.)

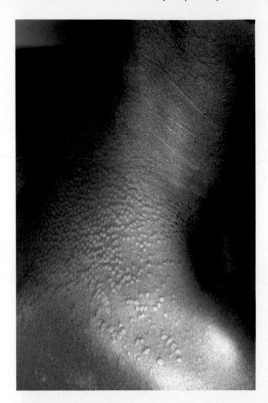

FIGURE 6-4. Perifollicular skin-colored papules on the upper mid-back extending onto the shoulders. The papular variant of pityriasis rosea is seen more commonly in people with skin of color. (Reproduced with permission from Taylor SC, Kelly AP, Lim HW, et al. *Taylor and Kelly's Dermatology for Skin of Color*, 2nd ed. New York, NY: McGraw Hill; 2016, Figure 25-8.)

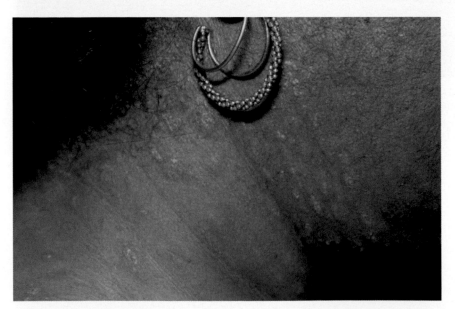

FIGURE 6-5. Another variant of pityriasis rosea is seen here as pink to pink-gray scaly plaques on the lateral neck, extending to the lateral jawline. (Reproduced with permission from Taylor SC, Kelly AP, Lim HW, et al. *Taylor and Kelly's Dermatology for Skin of Color*, 2nd ed. New York, NY: McGraw Hill; 2016, Figure 25-9B.)

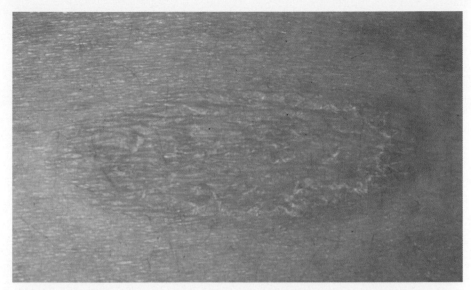

FIGURE 6-6. Pink to salmon-colored, oval-shaped, annular plaque with overlying trailing scale, which represents the classic presentation of a herald patch in lighter skin. (Reproduced with permission from Taylor SC, Kelly AP, Lim HW, et al. *Taylor and Kelly's Dermatology for Skin of Color*, 2nd ed. New York, NY: McGraw Hill; 2016, Figure 25-1A.)

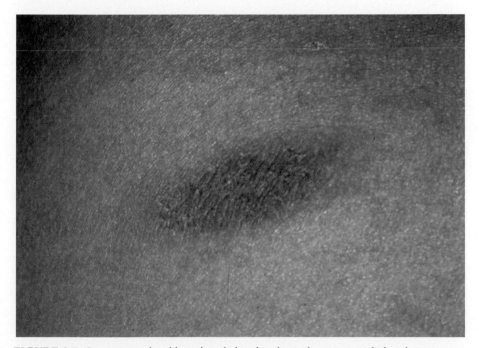

FIGURE 6-7. In contrast, a herald patch in darker skin shares the same morphology but varies in color. Seen here is a light red-purple, scaly, oval annular plaque that is lighter peripherally and darker centrally. (Reproduced with permission from Taylor SC, Kelly AP, Lim HW, et al. *Taylor and Kelly's Dermatology for Skin of Color*, 2nd ed. New York, NY: McGraw Hill; 2016, Figure 25-2A.)

KEY POINTS

- Seborrheic dermatitis can present with various presentations across skin colors including differences among those with darker skin.

- In individual with lighter skin, this condition typically presents with pink to bright-pink patches with overlying greasy scale in a seborrheic distribution that can include face, scalp, and trunk.

- Individuals with olive to light-brown skin can also have marked erythema signified by pink scaly hyperkeratotic patches. In darker brown skin, this may appear more hyperpigmented, brown to black, and scaly.

- Individuals with darker skin can also present with hypopigmented patches and plaques that lack significant scale in a seborrheic distribution, which can also signify active disease and can be misdiagnosed as vitiligo or postinflammatory hypopigmentation.

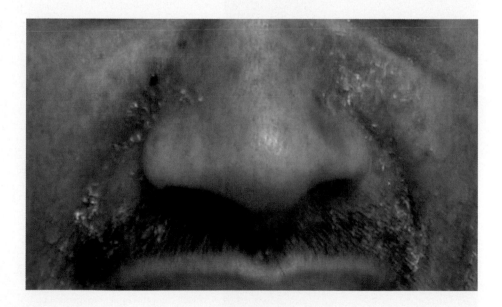

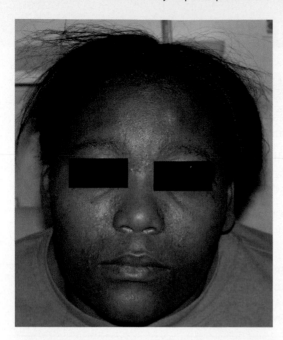

FIGURE 7-1. Brown scaly erythematous patches on glabella, mid-forehead, nasolabial folds, perioral area, and chin. (From Usatine RP, Smith MA, Mayeaux EJ Jr, et al. *The Color Atlas and Synopsis of Family Medicine*, 3rd ed. New York, NY: McGraw Hill; 2019, Figure 157-4. Reproduced with permission from Richard P. Usatine, MD.)

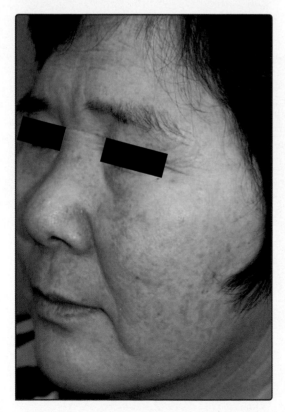

FIGURE 7-2. Bright-pink scaly patch seen along the left nasal ala, with scattered pink macules along the left cheek, chin, and upper cutaneous lip. (Reproduced with permission from Kang S, Amagai M, Bruckner AL, et al. *Fitzpatrick's Dermatology*, 9th ed. New York, NY: McGraw Hill; 2019, Figure 26-2B.)

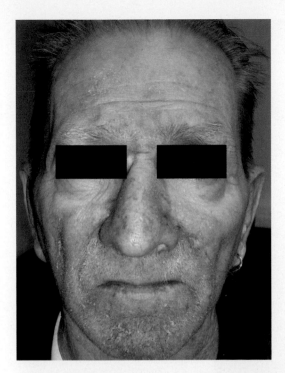

FIGURE 7-3. Generalized facial seborrheic dermatitis seen as pink patches with faint overlying scale involving the forehead, nose, cheeks, perioral skin, chin, and neck. Note the visible pink hue along eyelid margins. (From Usatine RP, Smith MA, Mayeaux EJ Jr, et al. *The Color Atlas and Synopsis of Family Medicine*, 3rd ed. New York, NY: McGraw Hill; 2019, Figure 157-1. Reproduced with permission from Richard P. Usatine, MD.)

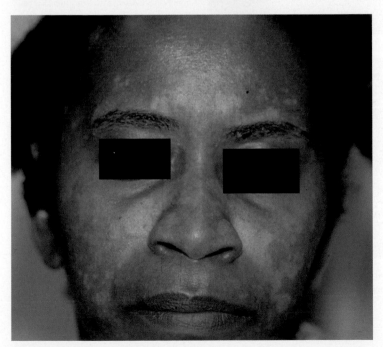

FIGURE 7-4. Marked hypopigmented patches along the nasal ala, nasolabial folds, cheeks, eyebrows, and forehead. Note the lack of significant overlying scale. (Reproduced with permission from Taylor SC, Kelly AP, Lim HW, et al. *Taylor and Kelly's Dermatology for Skin of Color*, 2nd ed. New York, NY: McGraw Hill; 2016, Figure 48-9.)

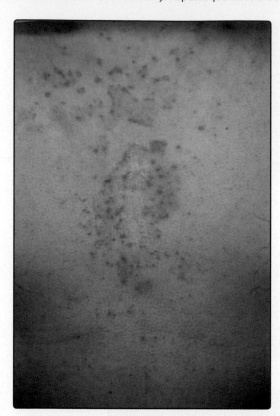

FIGURE 7-5. Diffuse scattered pink papules and macules overlying pink-brown patches on the chest, signifying postinflammatory change with minimal visible scale. (Reproduced with permission from Kang S, Amagai M, Bruckner AL, et al. *Fitzpatrick's Dermatology*, 9th ed. New York, NY: McGraw Hill; 2019, Figure 26-5.)

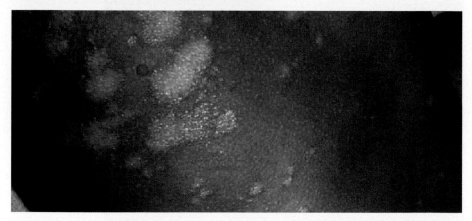

FIGURE 7-6. Multiple scattered, hypopigmented pink macules, patches, and plaques on the trunk. (Reproduced with permission from Burgin S. *Guidebook to Dermatologic Diagnosis*. New York, NY: McGraw Hill; 2021, Figure 12-12.)

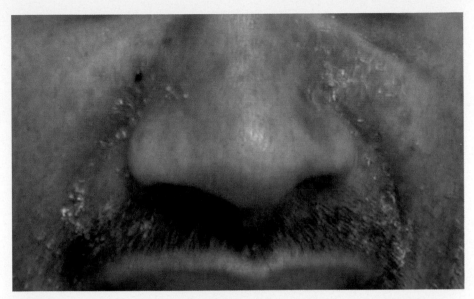

FIGURE 7-7. Bright-pink patches with overlying yellow hyperkeratotic scale on the bilateral nasolabial folds and upper cutaneous lip. Note the visible faint-pink macules on nose and infraorbital eyelids. (From Taylor SC, Kelly AP, Lim HW, et al. *Taylor and Kelly's Dermatology for Skin of Color*, 2nd ed. New York, NY: McGraw Hill; 2016, Figure 60-3. Reproduced with permission from the Ronald O. Perelman Department of Dermatology, NYU School of Medicine, NYU Langone Medical Center, NY.)

KEY POINTS

- Lichen planus is an inflammatory disorder that varies in clinical presentation across skin colors and also has numerous unique variants some of which are more common in darker skin populations.

- Classic lichen planus morphology in all skin colors tends to be flat, polygonal papules and plaques. However, the color varies and tends to be pink to red in lighter skin in contrast to the classic presentation in darker skin, which is typically purple to violaceous or brown to gray.

- Variants of lichen planus that can be seen more commonly in darker skin colors include annular, actinic, and follicular lichen planus.

- Lichen planus can also resolve with significant postinflammatory pigment alteration, particularly in those with darker skin.

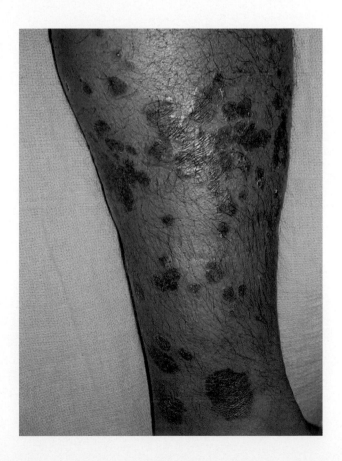

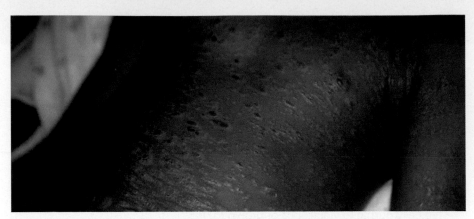

FIGURE 8-1. Flat-topped, purple, polygonal scaly papules on the trunk and posterior upper extremity. Note the gray-purple macules centrally, signifying resolving lesions of lichen planus. (Reproduced with permission from Burgin S: *Guidebook to Dermatologic Diagnosis*. New York, NY: McGraw Hill; 2021, Figure 4-11A.)

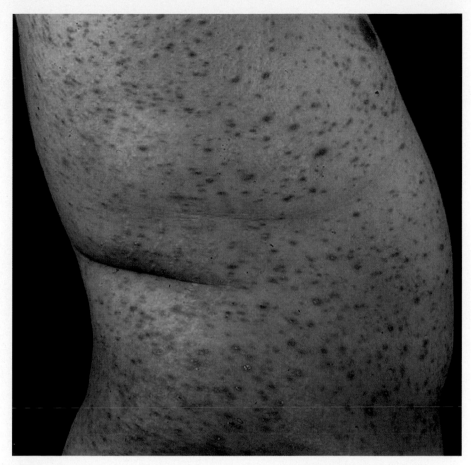

FIGURE 8-2. Red-maroon polymorphic papules scattered diffusely on the trunk. Note the overlying scale on the papules located on the lower lateral trunk. (Reproduced with permission from Wolff K, Johnson RA, Saavedra AP, Roh EK. *Fitzpatrick's Color Atlas and Synopsis of Clinical Dermatology,* 8th ed. New York, NY: McGraw Hill; 2017, Figure 14-17.)

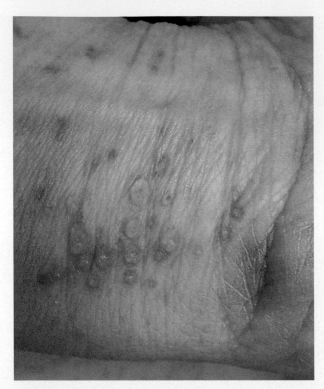

FIGURE 8-3. Pink, flat-topped, clustered papules lacking overlying scale on the ventral wrist. Not the pink-red macules inferior and lateral to the papules, signifying postinflammatory erythema from resolving lichen planus. (Reproduced with permission from Soutor C, Hordinsky MK. *Clinical Dermatology.* New York, NY: McGraw Hill; 2013, Figure 9-10.)

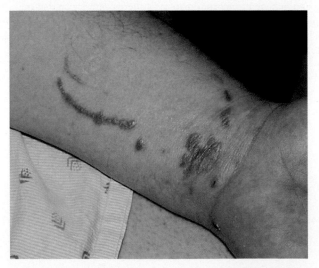

FIGURE 8-4. Red-purple polygonal flat-topped papules coalescing into plaques, one of which is linear, representing koebnerization. (Reproduced with permission from Soutor C, Hordinsky MK. *Clinical Dermatology.* New York, NY: McGraw Hill; 2013, Figure 9-11.)

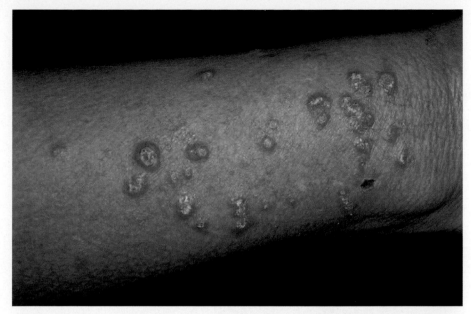

FIGURE 8-5. Discrete, pink-brown, polymorphic scaly papules on the forearm. (From Usatine RP, Smith MA, Mayeaux EJ Jr, Chumley HS. *The Color Atlas and Synopsis of Family Medicine*, 3rd ed. New York, NY: McGraw Hill; 2019, Figure 174-9. Reproduced with permission from Richard P. Usatine, MD.)

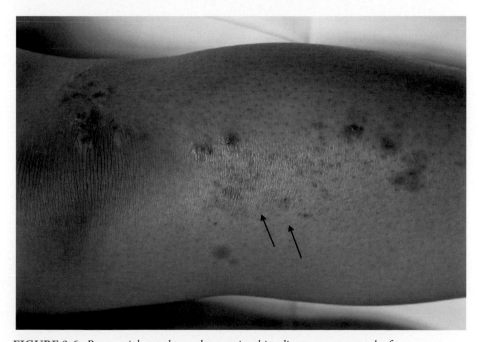

FIGURE 8-6. Brown-pink papules on the anterior shin adjacent to a gray patch of postinflammatory hyperpigmentation from resolving lichen planus. Note the variation in color, with several red-pink papules laterally and inferiorly on the shin. (Reproduced with permission from Burgin S: *Guidebook to Dermatologic Diagnosis*. New York, NY: McGraw Hill; 2021, Figure 3-28.)

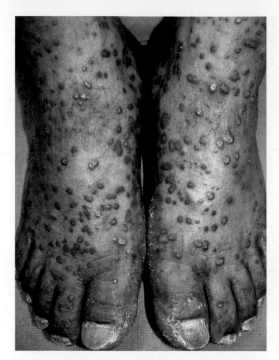

FIGURE 8-7. Numerous pink-purple papules, some with overlying scale, on the dorsal feet extending onto the dorsal toes. (From Usatine RP, Smith MA, Mayeaux EJ Jr, Chumley HS. *The Color Atlas and Synopsis of Family Medicine*, 3rd ed. New York, NY: McGraw Hill; 2019, Figure 160-17. Reproduced with permission from Eric Kraus, MD.)

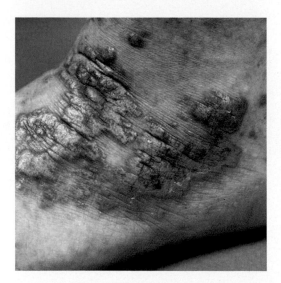

FIGURE 8-8. Maroon-white flat-topped plaques on the foot. In addition, on the foot there are also classic purple flat-topped papules of lichen planus. (Reproduced with permission from Wolff K, Johnson RA, Saavedra AP, Roh EK. *Fitzpatrick's Color Atlas and Synopsis of Clinical Dermatology*, 8th ed. New York, NY: McGraw Hill; 2017, Figure 14-16.)

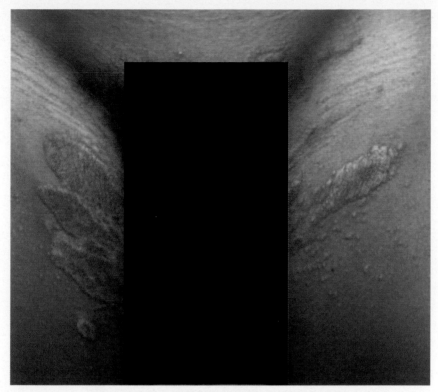

FIGURE 8-9. Dark-purple–black confluent plaques with pink periphery. (From Taylor SC, Kelly AP, Lim HW, Serrano AMA, eds. *Taylor and Kelly's Dermatology for Skin of Color*, 2nd ed. New York, NY: McGraw Hill; 2016, Figure 95-24. Used with permission from Dr. Marcia Ramos-e-Silva.)

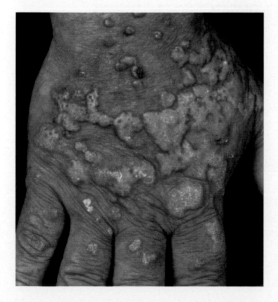

FIGURE 8-10. Pink-white flat-topped plaques on the dorsal hand. (Reproduced with permission from Wolff K, Johnson RA, Saavedra AP, Roh EK. *Fitzpatrick's Color Atlas and Synopsis of Clinical Dermatology*, 8th ed. New York, NY: McGraw Hill; 2017, Figure 14-16A.)

Actinic Lichen Planus

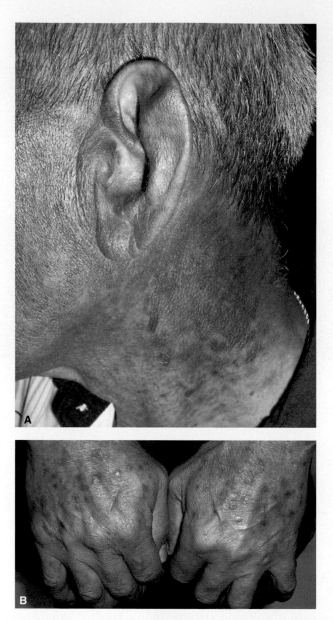

FIGURE 8-11. Black-gray papules and patches on the lateral face including ear and extending onto the neck (A) and similar morphology can be seen on the dorsal hands (B). Note the lack of overlying scale. (From Usatine RP, Smith MA, Mayeaux EJ Jr, Chumley HS. *The Color Atlas and Synopsis of Family Medicine*, 3rd ed. New York, NY: McGraw Hill; 2019, Figure 160-9. Reproduced with permission from Richard P. Usatine, MD.)

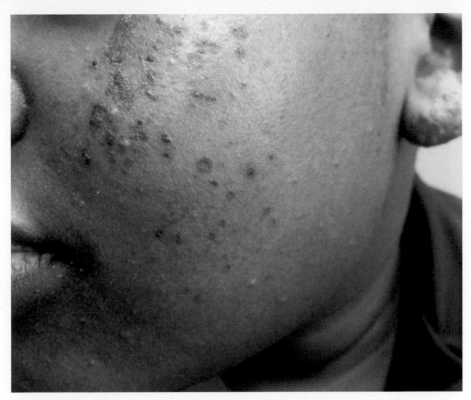

FIGURE 8-12. Purple-brown and black-brown fine papules along the left cheek and involving the left ear lobe. (Reproduced with permission from Prose NS, Kristal L. *Weinberg's Color Atlas of Pediatric Dermatology*, 5th ed. New York, NY: McGraw Hill; 2017, Figure 12-86.)

Annular Lichen Planus

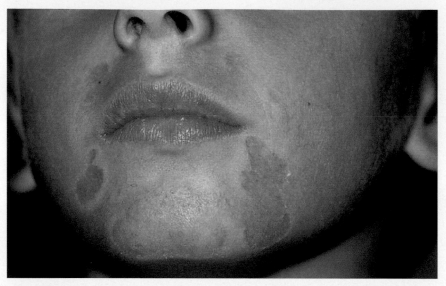

FIGURE 8-13. Discrete, annular, atrophic brown plaques with a rim of hypopigmentation on the face. (Reproduced with permission from Prose NS, Kristal L. *Weinberg's Color Atlas of Pediatric Dermatology*, 5th ed. New York, NY: McGraw Hill; 2017, Figure 12-87.)

Follicular Lichen Planus

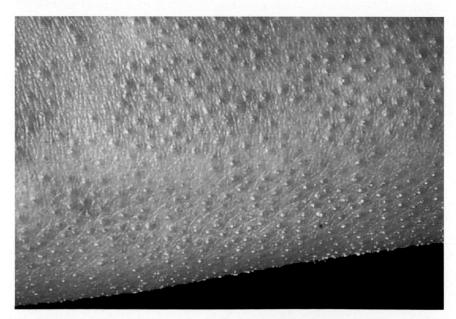

FIGURE 8-14. Numerous skin-colored perifollicular papules on an extremity. (Reproduced with permission from Prose NS, Kristal L. *Weinberg's Color Atlas of Pediatric Dermatology*, 5th ed. New York, NY: McGraw Hill; 2017, Figure 12-88.)

Hypertrophic Lichen Planus

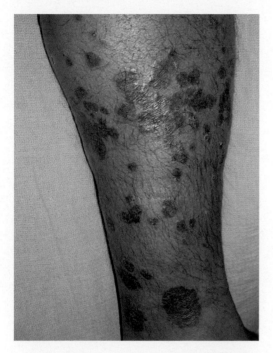

FIGURE 8-15. Numerous violaceous, flat-topped polygonal papules coalescing into plaques on the anterior shin. (From Usatine RP, Smith MA, Mayeaux EJ Jr, Chumley HS. *The Color Atlas and Synopsis of Family Medicine*, 3rd ed. New York, NY: McGraw Hill; 2019, Figure 160-7. Reproduced with permission from Richard P. Usatine, MD.)

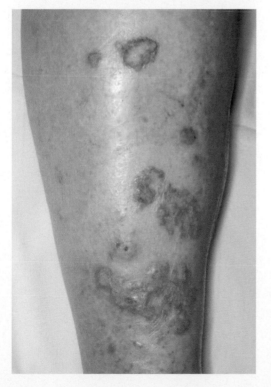

FIGURE 8-16. Pink-purple papules coalescing into plaques with an area of background peripheral brown pigmentation. (From Kang S, Amagai M, Bruckner AL, et al. *Fitzpatrick's Dermatology*, 9th ed. New York, NY: McGraw Hill; 2019, Figure 32-4. Used with permission from Mayo Foundation for Medical Education and Research, all rights reserved.)

KEY POINTS

- Lichen nitidus has a morphology of pinpoint to flat-topped papules that is similar across skin colors.

- However, the color of these papules can vary across skin colors from hypopigmented to skin colored to pink.

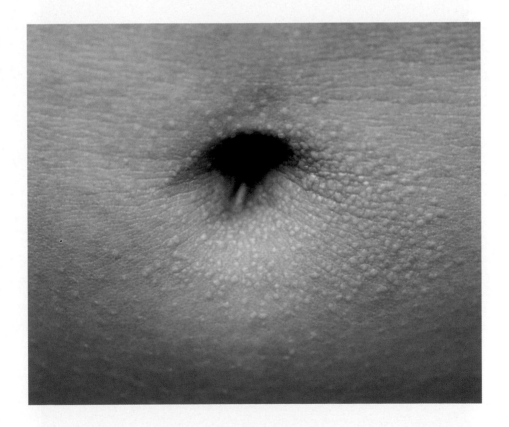

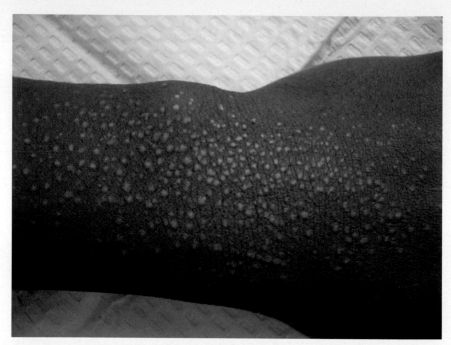

FIGURE 9-1. Numerous clustered light-brown to skin-colored fine monomorphic papules along the extensor forearm extending onto the dorsal hand. (Reproduced with permission from Kang S, Amagai M, Bruckner AL, et al. *Fitzpatrick's Dermatology*, 9th ed. New York, NY: McGraw Hill; 2019, Figure 1-3.)

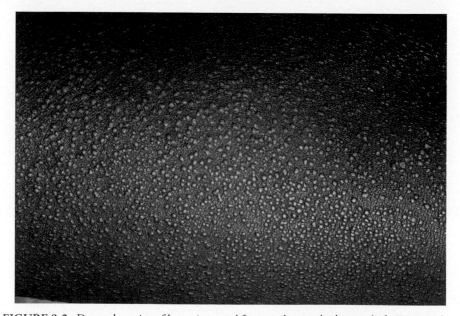

FIGURE 9-2. Dense clustering of hypopigmented fine papules on a background of a Fitzpatrick type VI person from Africa. (From Taylor SC, Kelly AP, Lim HW, et al. *Taylor and Kelly's Dermatology for Skin of Color*, 2nd ed. New York, NY: McGraw Hill; 2016, Figure 95-19. Reproduced with permission from Barbara Leppard.)

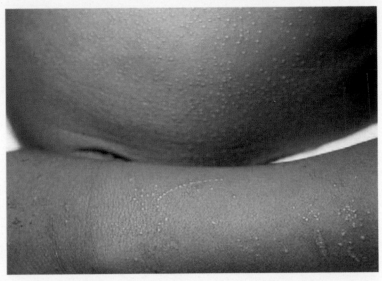

FIGURE 9-3. Scattered hypopigmented to skin-colored papules on the abdomen and arm, some of which are in a linear configuration representing koebnerization. (Reproduced with permission from Tilly JJ, Drolet BA, Esterly NB. Lichenoid eruptions in children. *J Am Acad Dermatol*, 2004;51(4):606-624.)

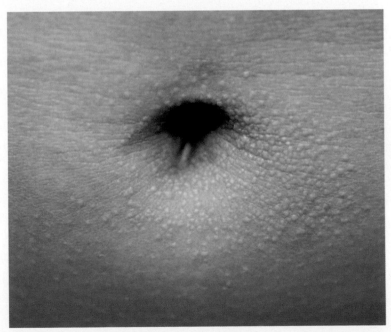

FIGURE 9-4. Periumbilical hypopigmented to skin-colored fine papules expanding centrifugally onto the abdomen, with areas of subtle background erythema. (Reproduced with permission from Prose NS, Kristal L. *Weinberg's Color Atlas of Pediatric Dermatology*, 5th ed. New York, NY: McGraw Hill; 2017, Figure 12-53.)

Infections

KEY POINTS

- Tinea versicolor can be localized or widespread and most commonly presents on the trunk but can also present on the face.

- In lighter skin types, it tends to present as pink to salmon-colored scaly patches, while in darker skin, it is also scaly but can vary in color from being hyperpigmented and gray to hypopigmented.

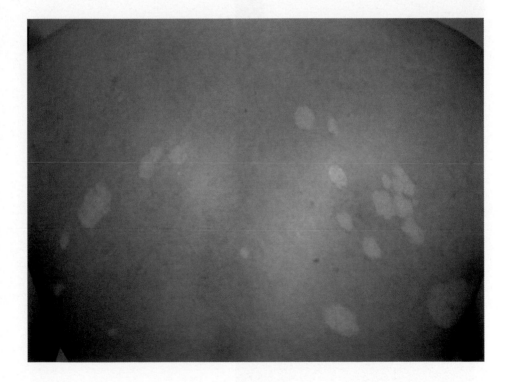

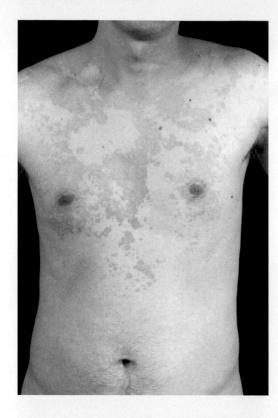

FIGURE 10-1. Tan macules and large patches on the anterior trunk of a White man. (Reproduced with permission from Wolff K, Johnson RA, Saavedra AP, et al. *Fitzpatrick's Color Atlas and Synopsis of Clinical Dermatology*, 8th ed. New York, NY: McGraw Hill; 2017, Figure 26-18.)

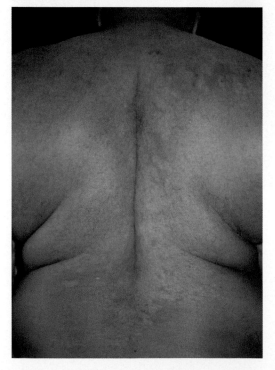

FIGURE 10-2. Hyperpigmented, gray, scaly confluent patches on the back of a Black man. (Reproduced with permission from Wolff K, Johnson RA, Saavedra AP, et al. *Fitzpatrick's Color Atlas and Synopsis of Clinical Dermatology*, 8th ed. New York, NY: McGraw Hill; 2017, Figure 26-20.)

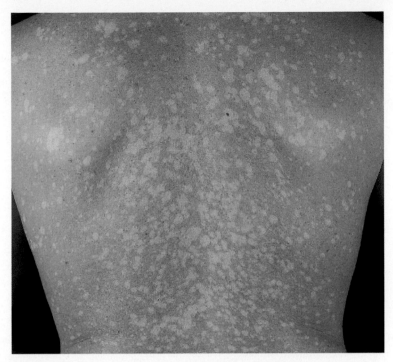

FIGURE 10-3. Diffuse hypopigmented macule and patches on the back of a White person. (Reproduced with permission from Wolff K, Johnson RA, Saavedra AP, et al. *Fitzpatrick's Color Atlas and Synopsis of Clinical Dermatology*, 8th ed. New York, NY: McGraw Hill; 2017, Figure 26-19.)

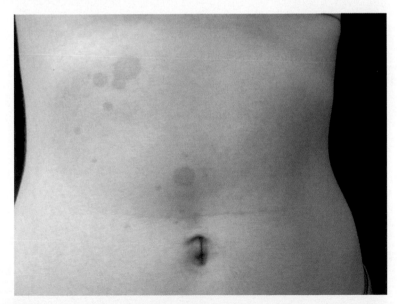

FIGURE 10-4. Nummular pink macules, patches, and plaques with minimal overlong scale on the anterior trunk. (Reproduced with permission from Kane KS, Nambudiri VE, Stratigos AJ. *Color Atlas & Synopsis of Pediatric Dermatology*, 3rd ed. New York, NY: McGraw Hill; 2017, Figure 21-17.)

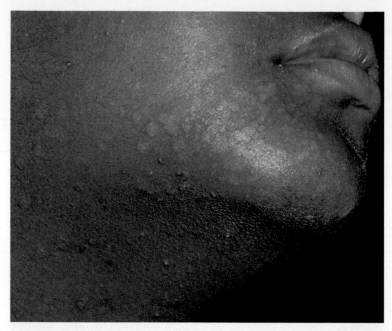

FIGURE 10-5. Small hypopigmented macules clustered along the chin and jawline. This location is a less common site for tinea versicolor. (Reproduced with permission from Prose NS, Kristal L. *Weinberg's Color Atlas of Pediatric Dermatology*, 5th ed. New York, NY: McGraw Hill; 2017, Figure 6-38.)

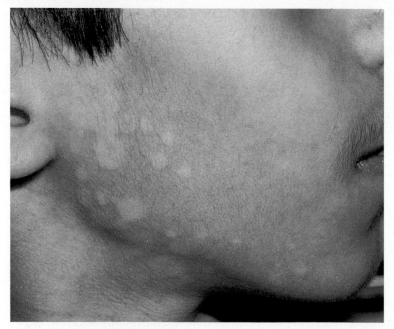

FIGURE 10-6. Hypopigmented macules along the jawline of a young person. (Reproduced with permission from Prose NS, Kristal L. *Weinberg's Color Atlas of Pediatric Dermatology*, 5th ed. New York, NY: McGraw Hill; 2017, Figure 6-40.)

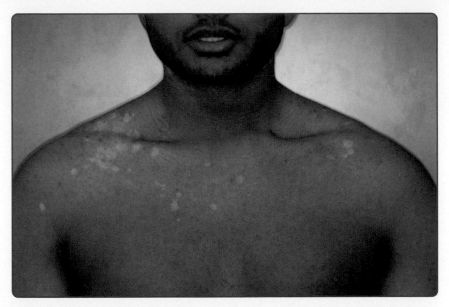

FIGURE 10-7. Hypopigmented macules coalescing into patches on the anterior trunk of a male with medium brown skin. (Reproduced with permission from Kang S, Amagai M, Bruckner AL, et al. *Fitzpatrick's Dermatology*, 9th ed. New York, NY: McGraw Hill; 2019, Figure 76-14.)

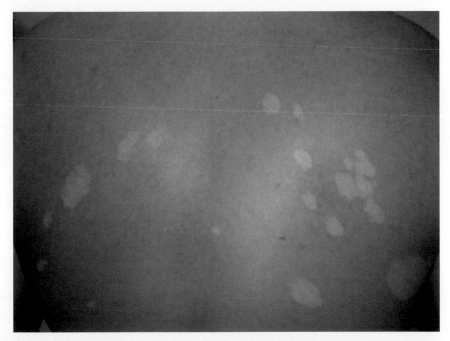

FIGURE 10-8. Hypopigmented patches on the back of a Latino man, which can be confused with other disorders of hypopigmentation and depigmentation, including hypopigmented mycosis fungoides and vitiligo, respectively. (From Usatine RP, Smith MA, Mayeaux EJ Jr, et al. *The Color Atlas and Synopsis of Family Medicine*, 3rd ed. New York, NY: McGraw Hill; 2019, Figure 147-2. Reproduced with permission from Richard P. Usatine, MD.)

KEY POINTS

- Tinea corporis can present with patches and plaques that may coalesce, and that are most commonly on the trunk and upper and lower extremities.

- In lighter skin, these patches and plaques are often pink to red in color and can have central pallor and a collarette of leading scale.

- In darker skin, these patches are also scaly and tend to be pink-brown to violaceous or gray in color. In some cases, the scale may be thick enough to obscure the underlying erythema or dyspigmentation.

- Resolving tinea corporis may also display areas of hyper- or hypopigmentation.

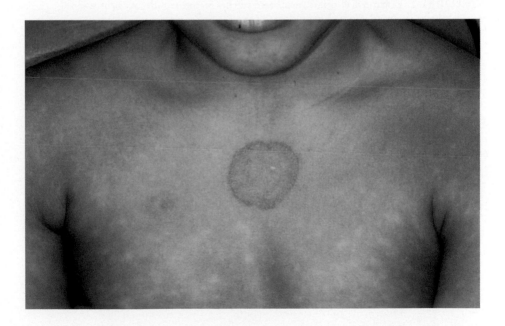

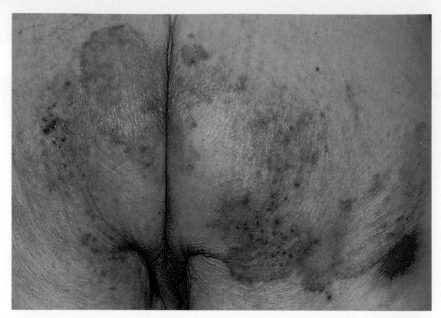

FIGURE 11-1. Bright-red, ill-defined excoriated patches on the buttocks of a light-skinned person who had been using topical steroids on the area, leading to tinea incognito. (Reproduced with permission from Wolff K, Johnson RA, Saavedra AP, et al. *Fitzpatrick's Color Atlas and Synopsis of Clinical Dermatology*, 8th ed. New York, NY: McGraw Hill; 2017, Figure 26-37.)

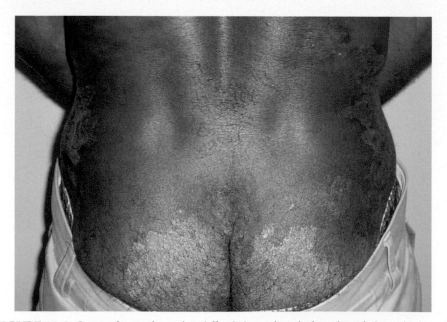

FIGURE 11-2. Large, silver, scaly patches diffusely located on the lateral trunk, lower back, and buttocks. Note the lack of erythema in this person with active disease. (From Usatine RP, Smith MA, Mayeaux EJ Jr, et al. *The Color Atlas and Synopsis of Family Medicine*, 3rd ed. New York, NY: McGraw Hill; 2019, Figure 144-3. Reproduced with permission from Richard P. Usatine, MD.)

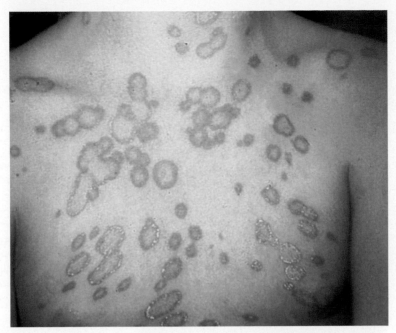

FIGURE 11-3. Numerous scattered, pink, nummular plaques with trailing scale and central clearing on the anterior neck and chest. (Reproduced with permission from Prose NS, Kristal L. *Weinberg's Color Atlas of Pediatric Dermatology*, 5th ed. New York, NY: McGraw Hill; 2017, Figure 6-5.)

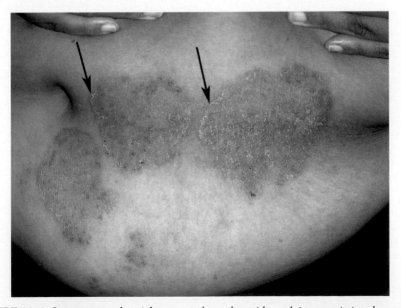

FIGURE 11-4. Large, nummular, violaceous, scaly patches with overlying excoriations located on that abdomen of a dark-skinned person. (From Usatine RP, Smith MA, Mayeaux EJ Jr, et al. *The Color Atlas and Synopsis of Family Medicine*, 3rd ed. New York, NY: McGraw Hill; 2019, Figure 215-5. Reproduced with permission from Richard P. Usatine, MD.)

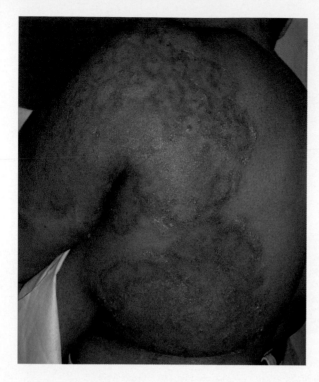

FIGURE 11-5. Large, annular, arcuate violaceous, and dark-brown patches and plaques with trailing scale located on the lateral trunk and posterior upper extremity. (From Burgin S: *Guidebook to Dermatologic Diagnosis*, New York, NY: McGraw Hill; 2021, Figure 6-35. Reproduced with permission from the Ronald O. Perelman Department of Dermatology, NYU School of Medicine, NYU Langone Medical Center, NY.)

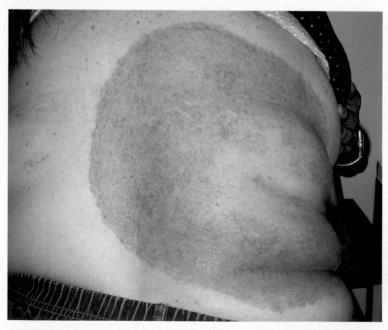

FIGURE 11-6. Large pink-brown patch with central clearing on the posterior trunk. (From Usatine RP, Smith MA, Mayeaux EJ Jr, et al. *The Color Atlas and Synopsis of Family Medicine*, 3rd ed. New York, NY: McGraw Hill; 2019, Figure 144-4. Reproduced with permission from Richard P. Usatine, MD.)

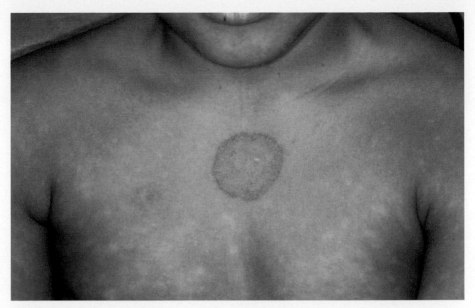

FIGURE 11-7. Red annular plaque with central clearing on the mid-chest of a dark-skinned person. Note the surrounding hypopigmented macules and patches secondary to resolved tinea corporis. (Reproduced with permission from Barnhill RL, Crowson AN, Magro CM, et al. *Barnhill's Dermatopathology*, 4th ed. New York, NY: McGraw Hill; 2020, Figure 21-1A.)

KEY POINTS

- Cellulitis is an infectious process that carries the risk for sepsis if not treated in a timely manner.

- In lighter skin, it tends to be bright red and well demarcated and can have accompanying signs of warmth and tenderness.

- In darker skin, cellulitis can be violaceous to dusky gray and more subtle with significant masking of the erythema, which can lead to risk of missed or delayed diagnoses.

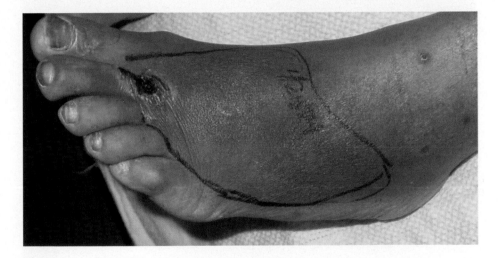

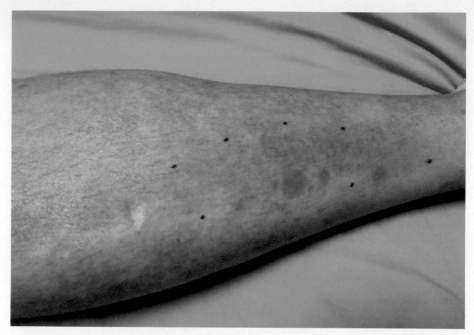

FIGURE 12-1. Brown to pink patch along the lateral shin of a dark-skinned person. Note the subtlety of the erythema more proximally on the leg. (Reproduced with permission from Kang S, Amagai M, Bruckner AL, et al. *Fitzpatrick's Dermatology*, 9th ed. New York, NY: McGraw Hill; 2019, Figure 151-1.)

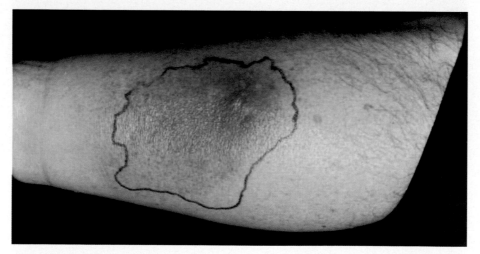

FIGURE 12-2. Bright-red edematous patch along the shin of the lower extremity. (Reproduced with permission from Wolff K, Johnson RA, Saavedra AP, et al. *Fitzpatrick's Color Atlas and Synopsis of Clinical Dermatology*, 8th ed. New York, NY: McGraw Hill; 2017, Figure 25-27.)

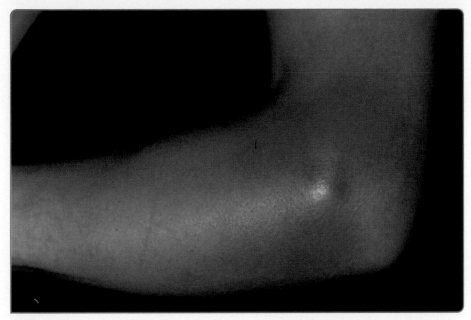

FIGURE 12-3. Deep-red edematous patch extending along the upper extremity. (Reproduced with permission from Kang S, Amagai M, Bruckner AL, et al. *Fitzpatrick's Dermatology*, 9th ed. New York, NY: McGraw Hill; 2019, Figure 151-2B.)

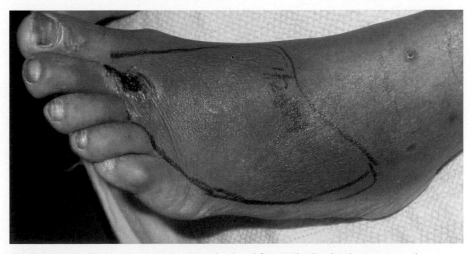

FIGURE 12-4. Pink-violaceous plaque on the dorsal foot, with a localized gangrenous plaque at the base of the second dorsal digit in a person with diabetes. (From Usatine RP, Smith MA, Mayeaux EJ Jr, et al. *The Color Atlas and Synopsis of Family Medicine*, 3rd ed. New York, NY: McGraw Hill; 2019, Figure 126-3. Reproduced with permission from Richard P. Usatine, MD.)

KEY POINTS

- Secondary syphilis can present with varying morphologies including macular, papular, papulosquamous, and annular plaques across skin colors.

- On acral surfaces in lighter skin, it is often bright pink to red, while in darker skin, it tends to be brown to violaceous. Overlying scale may or may not be present.

- On nonacral surfaces, in lighter skin, it tends to be pink to red, while in darker skin, it can be pink to brown to violaceous. Additionally, the annular variant can also have a hypopigmented peripheral rim.

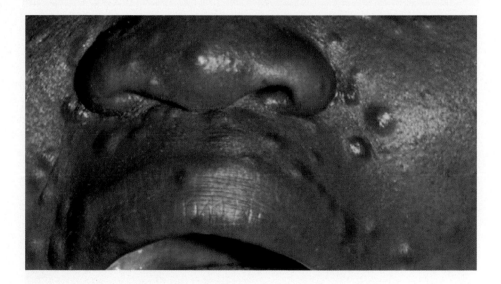

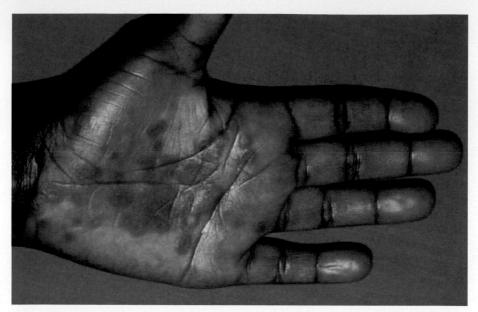

FIGURE 13-1. Violaceous papules coalescing centrally into plaques on the left palmar hand. (Reproduced with permission from Soutor C, Hordinsky MK. *Clinical Dermatology*. New York, NY: McGraw Hill; 2013, Figure 1-8A.)

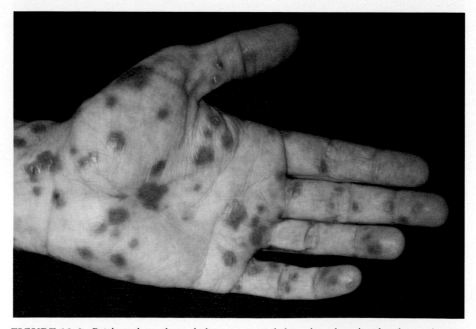

FIGURE 13-2. Bright-red papules and plaques scattered along the palmar hand and ventral wrist. (From Usatine RP, Smith MA, Mayeaux EJ Jr, et al. *The Color Atlas and Synopsis of Family Medicine*, 3rd ed. New York, NY: McGraw Hill; 2019, Figure 225-15B. Reproduced with permission from Jonathan B. Karnes, MD.)

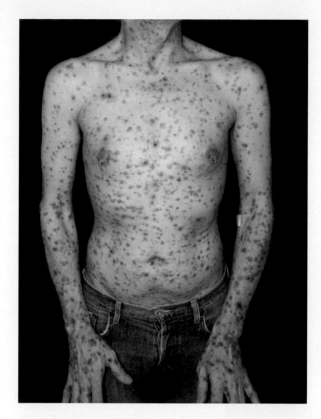

FIGURE 13-3. Diffuse red papules and plaques on the neck, trunk, and upper extremities. (From Usatine RP, Smith MA, Mayeaux EJ Jr, et al. *The Color Atlas and Synopsis of Family Medicine*, 3rd ed. New York, NY: McGraw Hill; 2019, Figure 225-15A. Reproduced with permission from Jonathan B. Karnes, MD.)

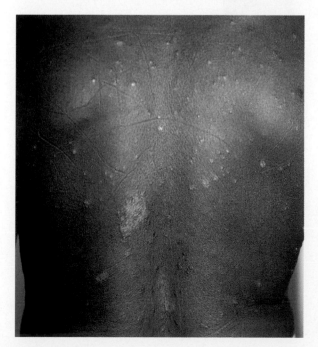

FIGURE 13-4. Pink scaly papules and plaques of varying sizes scattered diffusely along the back. Note the dark-brown patches along the mid-lower and lateral back signifying postinflammatory changes. (Reproduced with permission from Soutor C, Hordinsky MK. *Clinical Dermatology*. New York, NY: McGraw Hill; 2013, Figure 12-6.)

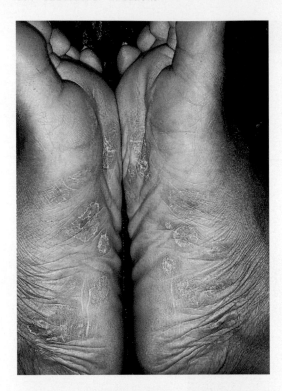

FIGURE 13-5. Brown plaques with overlying silvery-white scale along the bilateral planter feet. (Reproduced with permission from Wolff K, Johnson RA, Saavedra AP, et al. *Fitzpatrick's Color Atlas and Synopsis of Clinical Dermatology*, 8th ed. New York, NY: McGraw Hill; 2017, Figure 30-31.)

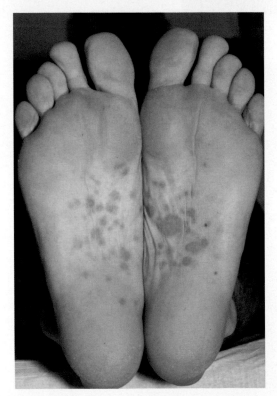

FIGURE 13-6. Salmon-colored macules and patches on the bilateral plantar feet. (Reproduced with permission from Barnhill RL, Crowson AN, Magro CM, et al. *Barnhill's Dermatopathology*, 4th ed. New York, NY: McGraw Hill; 2020, Figure 20-4A.)

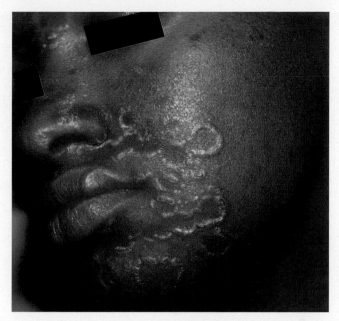

FIGURE 13-7. Annular violaceous plaques with lighter pink raised borders on the face of a Latin American person. (From Taylor SC, Kelly AP, Lim HW, et al. *Taylor and Kelly's Dermatology for Skin of Color*, 2nd ed. New York, NY: McGraw Hill; 2016, Figure 95-57. Reproduced with permission from Parish LC, Brenner S, Ramos-e-Silva M, et al. *Atlas of Women's Dermatology*. London, United Kingdom: Taylor & Francis; 2006.)

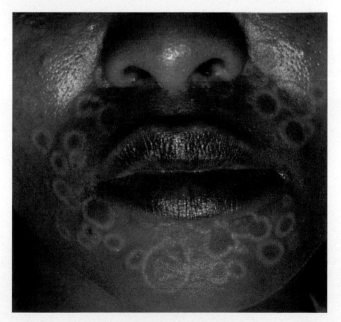

FIGURE 13-8. Dark-brown plaques with hypopigmented raised borders on the perioral skin of a South African woman. (From Wolff K, Johnson RA, Saavedra AP, et al. *Fitzpatrick's Color Atlas and Synopsis of Clinical Dermatology*, 8th ed. New York, NY: McGraw Hill; 2017, Figure 30-32. Reproduced with permission from Jeffrey S. Dover, MD.)

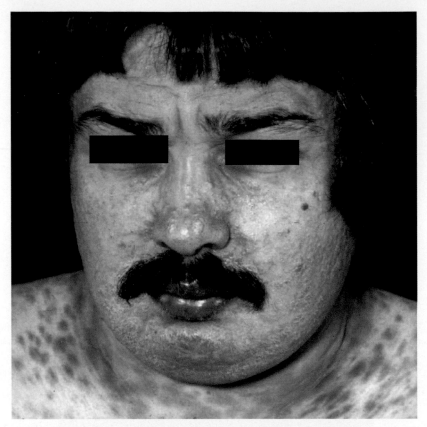

FIGURE 13-9. Fine pink papules overlying a background of erythema most notable along the nose and medial cheeks. (Reproduced with permission from Wolff K, Johnson RA, Saavedra AP, et al. *Fitzpatrick's Color Atlas and Synopsis of Clinical Dermatology*, 8th ed. New York, NY: McGraw Hill; 2017, Figure 30-29.)

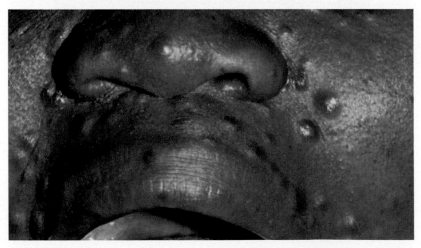

FIGURE 13-10. Violaceous and brown papules densely scattered along the nose, medial cheeks, and lips. (Reproduced with permission from Soutor C, Hordinsky MK. *Clinical Dermatology*. New York, NY: McGraw Hill; 2013, Figure 13-30.)

KEY POINTS

- The morphology of a verruca and condyloma tends to present as papules and/or plaques.

- On lighter skin, this can be pink to skin colored.

- In darker skin, it can present as pink-grey, pink-brown, brown, hypopigmented, or skin colored.

VERRUCA PLANA

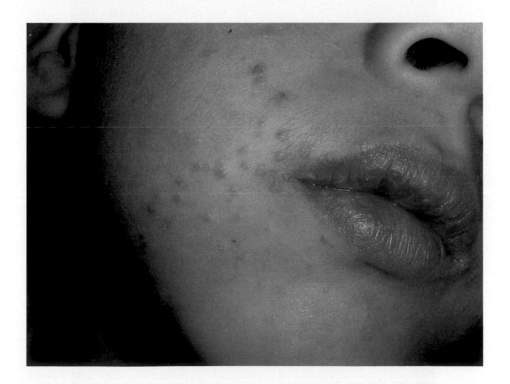

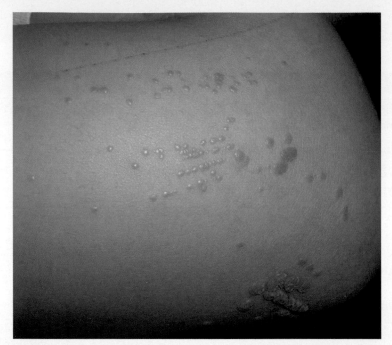

FIGURE 14-1. Pink and skin-colored papules of varying sizes on the upper extremity. Note the linear presentation of the skin-colored papules signifying koebnerization of the verruca. (From Usatine RP, Smith MA, Mayeaux EJ Jr, et al. *The Color Atlas and Synopsis of Family Medicine*, 3rd ed. New York, NY: McGraw Hill; 2019, Figure 138-4. Reproduced with permission from Richard P. Usatine, MD.)

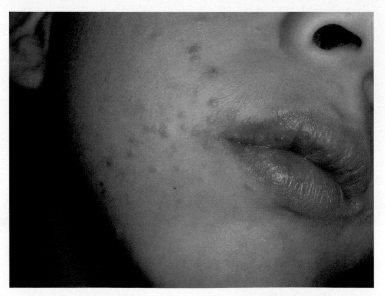

FIGURE 14-2. Multiple pink to skin-colored small papules along the left cheek and oral commissure. (From Usatine RP, Smith MA, Mayeaux EJ Jr, et al. *The Color Atlas and Synopsis of Family Medicine*, 3rd ed. New York, NY: McGraw Hill; 2019, Figure 138-5. Reproduced with permission from Richard P. Usatine, MD.)

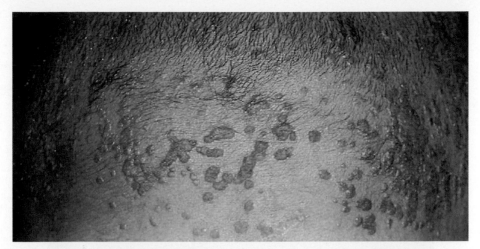

FIGURE 14-3. Brown discrete and clustered papules and plaques along the forehead of an immunosuppressed child. (Reproduced with permission from Wolff K, Johnson RA, Saavedra AP, et al. *Fitzpatrick's Color Atlas and Synopsis of Clinical Dermatology*, 8th ed. New York, NY: McGraw Hill; 2017, Figure 27-17.)

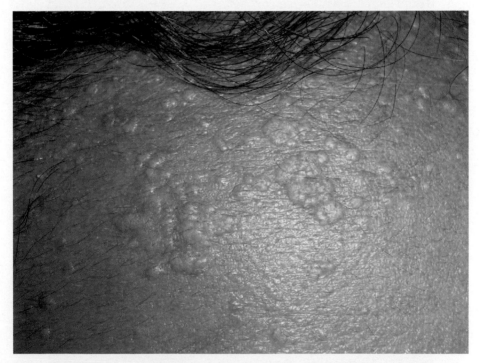

FIGURE 14-4. Light-pink papules and plaques scattered along the forehead. (From Usatine RP, Smith MA, Mayeaux EJ Jr, et al. *The Color Atlas and Synopsis of Family Medicine*, 3rd ed. New York, NY: McGraw Hill; 2019, Figure 138-1. Reproduced with permission from Richard P. Usatine, MD.)

VERRUCA VULGARIS

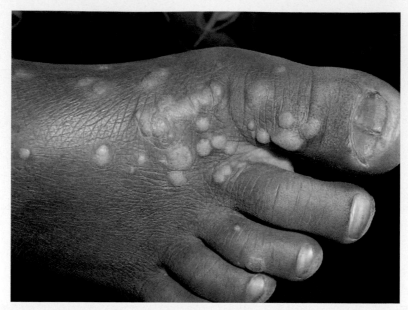

FIGURE 14-5. Multiple tan papules, several of which are coalescing into plaques located on the dorsal foot of a young immunosuppressed child. (From Usatine RP, Smith MA, Mayeaux EJ Jr, et al. *The Color Atlas and Synopsis of Family Medicine*, 3rd ed. New York, NY: McGraw Hill; 2019, Figure 137-4. Reproduced with permission from Richard P. Usatine, MD.)

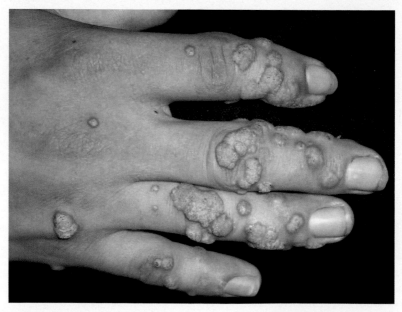

FIGURE 14-6. Pink hyperkeratotic papules and plaques along the dorsal hand. (From Usatine RP, Smith MA, Mayeaux EJ Jr, et al. *The Color Atlas and Synopsis of Family Medicine*, 3rd ed. New York, NY: McGraw Hill; 2019, Figure 137-2. Reproduced with permission from Richard P. Usatine, MD.)

CONDYLOMA

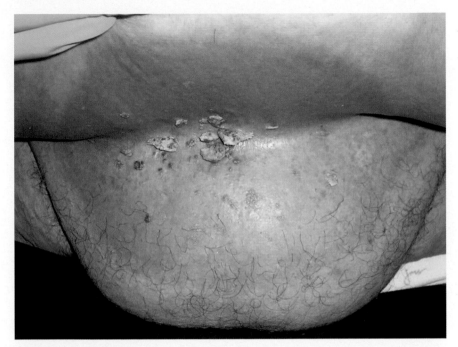

FIGURE 14-7. Pink to red macerated papules and plaques clustered on the pannus of an obese woman. (From Usatine RP, Smith MA, Mayeaux EJ Jr, et al. *The Color Atlas and Synopsis of Family Medicine*, 3rd ed. New York, NY: McGraw Hill; 2019, Figure 139-9. Reproduced with permission from Richard P. Usatine, MD.)

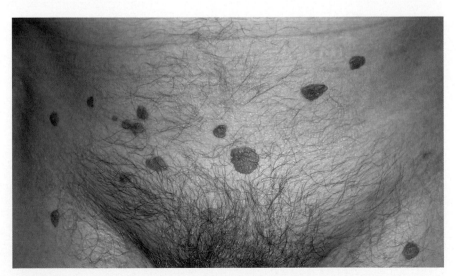

FIGURE 14-8. Large dark-brown papules on the suprapubic skin of a Latino man. (From Usatine RP, Smith MA, Mayeaux EJ Jr, et al. *The Color Atlas and Synopsis of Family Medicine*, 3rd ed. New York, NY: McGraw Hill; 2019, Figure 139-8. Reproduced with permission from Richard P. Usatine, MD.)

KEY POINTS

- Molluscum presents with small- to medium-size umbilicated papules across skin types.

- Papules can vary in color from pink and pearly in lighter skin to skin colored, hypopigmented, or pink-brown in dark skin.

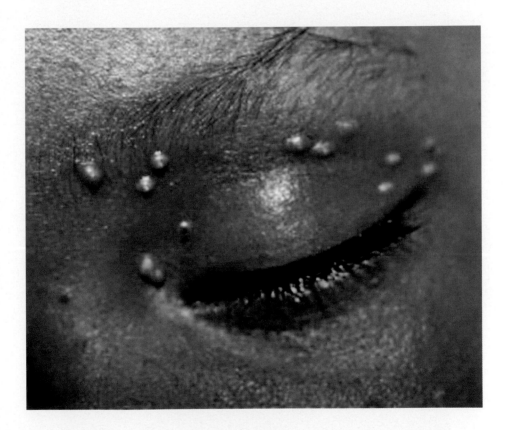

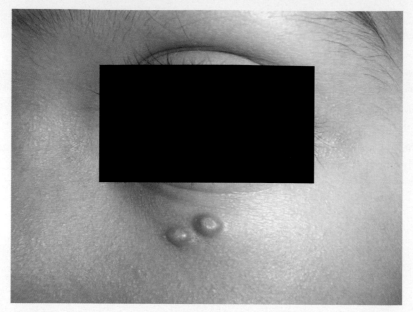

FIGURE 15-1. Pink to skin-colored discrete umbilicated papules on the lower eyelid. (From Usatine RP, Smith MA, Mayeaux EJ Jr, et al. *The Color Atlas and Synopsis of Family Medicine*, 3rd ed. New York, NY: McGraw Hill; 2019, Figure 136-4. Reproduced with permission from Richard P. Usatine, MD.)

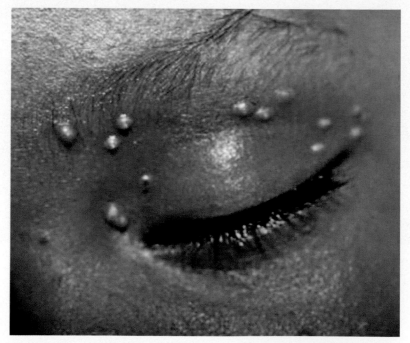

FIGURE 15-2. Skin-colored umbilicated papules scattered on the upper eyelid. (Reproduced with permission from Prose NS, Kristal L. *Weinberg's Color Atlas of Pediatric Dermatology*, 5th ed. New York, NY: McGraw Hill; 2017, Figure 5-2.)

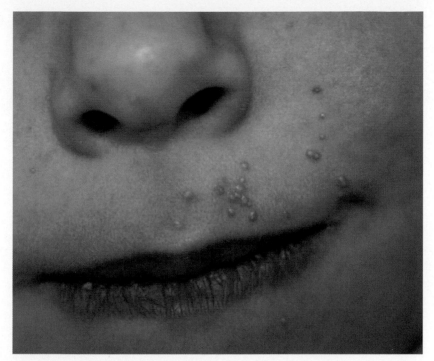

FIGURE 15-3. Clustered pink to skin-colored umbilicated papules on the upper cutaneous lip. (Reproduced with permission from Prose NS, Kristal L. *Weinberg's Color Atlas of Pediatric Dermatology*, 5th ed. New York, NY: McGraw Hill; 2017, Figure 5-3.)

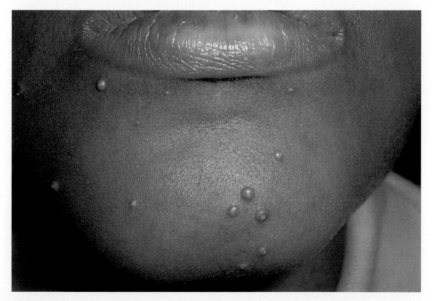

FIGURE 15-4. Umbilicated skin-colored discrete papules with white centers located on the chin of a young girl. (From Usatine RP, Smith MA, Mayeaux EJ Jr, et al. *The Color Atlas and Synopsis of Family Medicine*, 3rd ed. New York, NY: McGraw Hill; 2019, Figure 136-1. Reproduced with permission from Richard P. Usatine, MD.)

KEY POINTS

- Herpes simplex and varicella zoster both present with vesicular and papular morphologies that are often clustered and can become secondarily impetiginized.

- In lighter skin, this is often bright pink to red and can become darker centrally as it resolves.

- In darker skin, this can appear red to red-brown, violaceous, or skin-colored. Resolution in darker skin at the base of the vesicles is often dark brown.

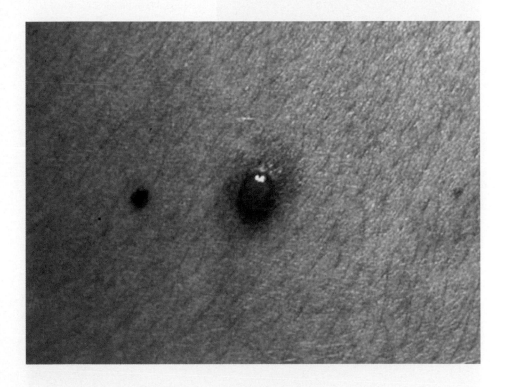

ECZEMA HERPETICUM

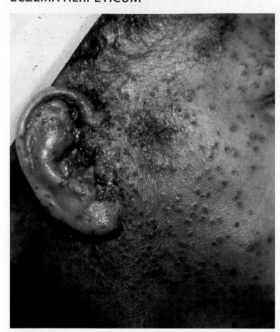

FIGURE 16-1. Pink monomorphic eroded papules densely scattered on the lateral face, with impetiginization visible along the ear. (Reproduced with permission from Burgin S. *Guidebook to Dermatologic Diagnosis*. New York, NY: McGraw Hill; 2021, Figure 8-22.)

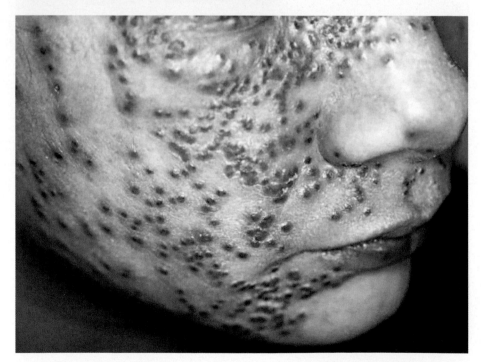

FIGURE 16-2. Pink-red eroded impetiginized papules densely scattered on the right side of the face. Note the amount of visible erythema surrounding each of these papules, which is less visible in the person with skin of color. (Reproduced with permission from Burgin S. *Guidebook to Dermatologic Diagnosis*. New York, NY: McGraw Hill; 2021, Figure 7-6).

HERPES SIMPLEX

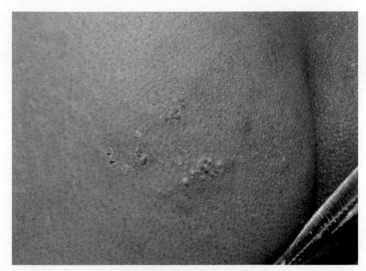

FIGURE 16-3. Pink clustered vesicles and pustules on an erythematous base of the left buttock representing active herpes simplex virus (HSV) infection. Superior to this are areas of resolving HSV infection, visible by the crusted violaceous papules surrounded by postinflammatory hyperpigmentation. (From Usatine RP, Smith MA, Mayeaux EJ Jr, et al. *The Color Atlas and Synopsis of Family Medicine*, 3rd ed. New York, NY: McGraw Hill; 2019, Figure 135-11. Reproduced with permission from Richard P. Usatine, MD.)

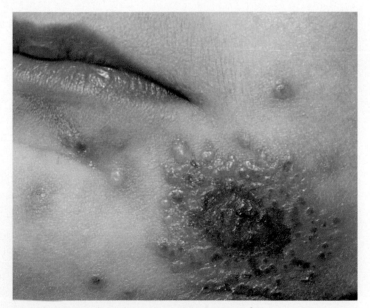

FIGURE 16-4. Pink grouped vesicles with central erosions and crusting in the perioral region of the face. (Reproduced with permission from Prose NS, Kristal L. *Weinberg's Color Atlas of Pediatric Dermatology*, 5th ed. New York, NY: McGraw Hill; 2017, Figure 5-36.)

VARICELLA ZOSTER

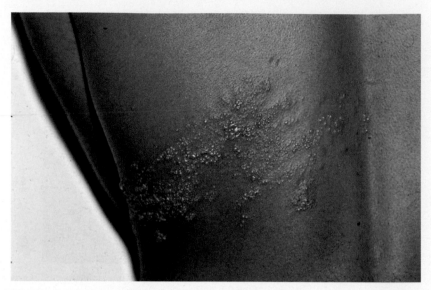

FIGURE 16-5. Light-brown to violaceous pinpoint vesicles coalescing into plaques, with a mild background of subtle pink erythema clustered along the thoracic dermatome. (Reproduced with permission from Burgin S. *Guidebook to Dermatologic Diagnosis.* New York, NY: McGraw Hill; 2021, Figure 7-8.)

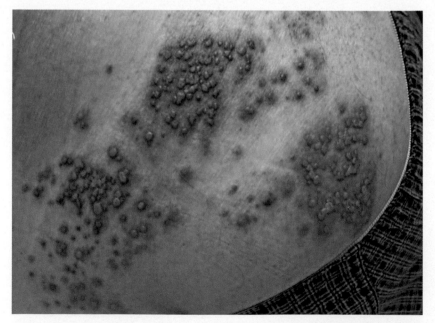

FIGURE 16-6. Bright-pink grouped vesicles coalescing into plaques with an intensely visible background of erythema. (Reproduced with permission from Burgin S, et al. *Guidebook to Dermatologic Diagnosis.* New York, NY: McGraw Hill; 2021, Figure 2-41.)

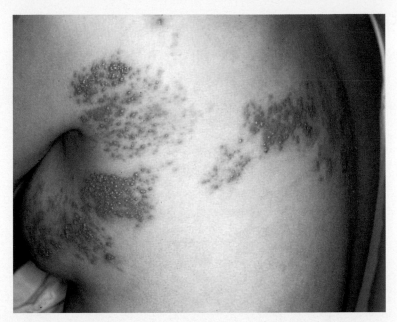

FIGURE 16-7. Multiple plaques of grouped vesicles on an erythematous base extending along the thoracic dermatome. (Reproduced with permission from Soutor C, Hordinsky MK. *Clinical Dermatology.* New York, NY: McGraw Hill; 2013, Figure 11-3.)

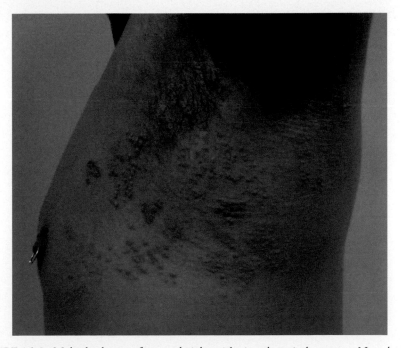

FIGURE 16-8. Multiple plaques of grouped pink vesicles in a thoracic dermatome. Note that the background of the vesicles in this patient is both erythematous and violaceous. (Reproduced with permission from Taylor SC, Kelly AP, Lim HW, et al. *Taylor and Kelly's Dermatology for Skin of Color*, 2nd ed. New York, NY: McGraw Hill; 2016, Figure 61-2.)

VARICELLA ZOSTER VIRUS

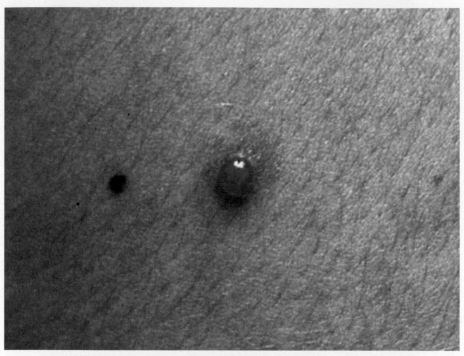

FIGURE 16-9. Bright-pink vesicle on an erythematous base representing a "dew drop on a rose petal." (From Usatine RP, Smith MA, Mayeaux EJ Jr, et al. *The Color Atlas and Synopsis of Family Medicine*, 3rd ed. New York, NY: McGraw Hill; 2019, Figure 129-5. Reproduced with permission from Richard P. Usatine, MD.)

KEY POINTS

- Scabies presents with a papular and vesicular morphology on all skin types that can vary most prominently in color.

- In darker skin, it can appear brown to violaceous in contrast to pink to skin colored in lighter skin.

- Darker skin can also have significant background hyperpigmentation that can be part of the active disease or postinflammatory in nature.

- In crusted scabies, the degree of hyperkeratosis can vary, and in darker skin, this may be extensive enough to mask any underlying erythema.

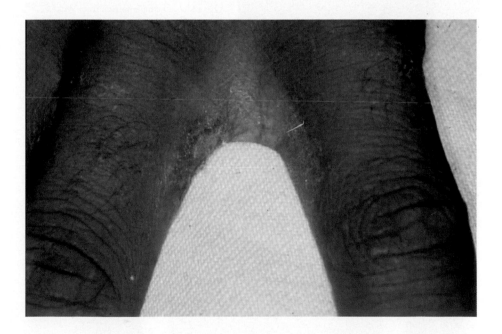

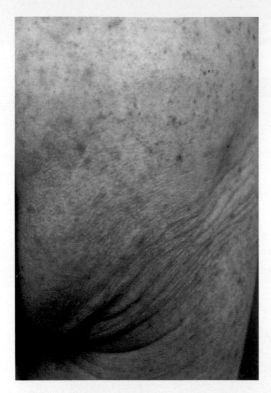

FIGURE 17-1. Diffuse pink papules and patches with overlying excoriations on the buttock of a middle-aged woman. (Reproduced with permission from Wolff K, Johnson RA, Saavedra AP, et al. *Fitzpatrick's Color Atlas and Synopsis of Clinical Dermatology*, 8th ed. New York, NY: McGraw Hill; 2017, Figure 28-23.)

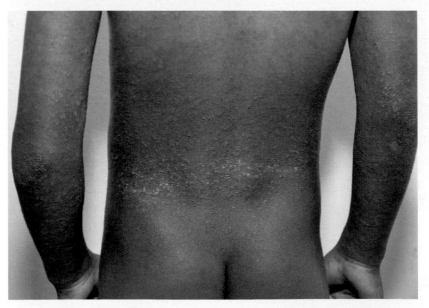

FIGURE 17-2. Diffuse dark-brown and skin-colored papules with areas of overlying scale and a background of hyperpigmentation on the trunk, buttocks, and posterior upper extremities. (From Usatine RP, Smith MA, Mayeaux EJ Jr, et al. *The Color Atlas and Synopsis of Family Medicine*, 3rd ed. New York, NY: McGraw Hill; 2019, Figure 149-16. Reproduced with permission from Richard P. Usatine, MD.)

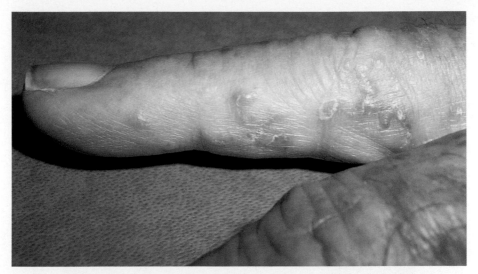

FIGURE 17-3. Pink papules, vesicles, and burrows on a digit. (From Usatine RP, Smith MA, Mayeaux EJ Jr, et al. *The Color Atlas and Synopsis of Family Medicine*, 3rd ed. New York, NY: McGraw Hill; 2019, Figure 149-11. Reproduced with permission from Richard P. Usatine, MD.)

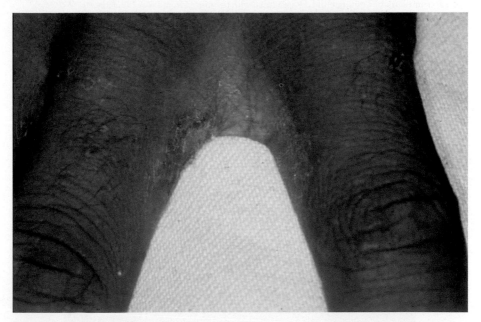

FIGURE 17-4. Pink scaly crusting and resolving vesicles in the interdigital webspace. (Reproduced with permission from Taylor SC, Kelly AP, Lim HW, et al. *Taylor and Kelly's Dermatology for Skin of Color*, 2nd ed. New York, NY: McGraw Hill; 2016, Figure 64-3.)

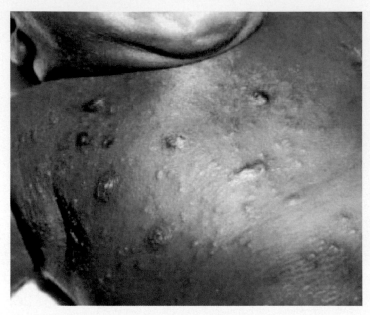

FIGURE 17-5. Scattered scaly violaceous nodules with surrounding pink papules in the axilla and the anterior trunk of a young child. (Reproduced with permission from Prose NS, Kristal L. *Weinberg's Color Atlas of Pediatric Dermatology*, 5th ed. New York, NY: McGraw Hill; 2017, Figure 8-17.)

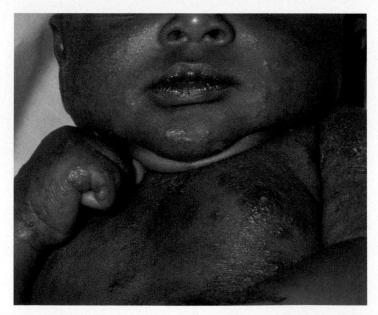

FIGURE 17-6. Pink, brown, and violaceous papules and plaques scattered along the face, chest, and upper extremities of an African infant. Note the variation in the colors of the papules, ranging from pink to erythematous on the face to violaceous and dark brown on the trunk and extremities. (From Taylor SC, Kelly AP, Lim HW, et al. *Taylor and Kelly's Dermatology for Skin of Color*, 2nd ed. New York, NY: McGraw Hill; 2016, Figure 95-52. Reproduced with permission from Barbara Leppard.)

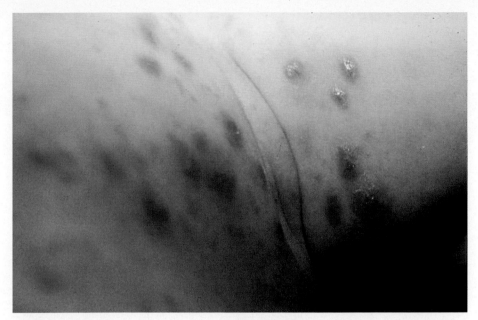

FIGURE 17-7. Bright-red papules with surrounding erythema and some with overlying scale on the lateral trunk of an infant with White skin. (Reproduced with permission from Kane KS, Nambudiri VE, Stratigos AJ. *Color Atlas & Synopsis of Pediatric Dermatology*, 3rd ed. New York, NY: McGraw Hill; 2017, Figure 25-6.)

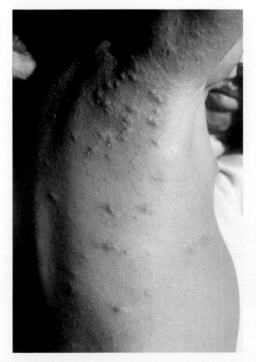

FIGURE 17-8. Diffuse skin-colored and light-brown papules and nodules, some of which have overlying scale and burrows on the lateral trunk and upper extremity of an 18-month-old child. (From Taylor SC, Kelly AP, Lim HW, et al. *Taylor and Kelly's Dermatology for Skin of Color*, 2nd ed. New York, NY: McGraw Hill; 2016, Figure 95-54. Reproduced with permission from Dr. Marcia Ramos-e-Silva.)

CRUSTED SCABIES

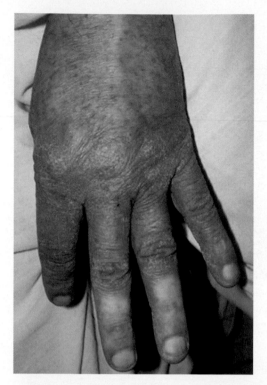

FIGURE 17-9. Yellow crusted plaques over the metacarpophalangeal and distal interphalangeal joints, with a background of erythema on the dorsal hand. (From Taylor SC, Kelly AP, Lim HW, et al. *Taylor and Kelly's Dermatology for Skin of Color*, 2nd ed. New York, NY: McGraw Hill; 2016, Figure 60-7. Reproduced with from the Ronald O. Perelman Department of Dermatology, NYU School of Medicine, NYU Langone Medical Center, NY.)

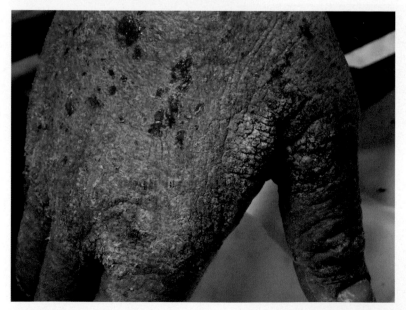

FIGURE 17-10. Hyperkeratotic crusted plaque covering the majority of the dorsal hand, with limited areas of sparing. (Reproduced with permission from Aiempanakit K. Crusted scabies in a patient with methamphetamine abuse. *JAAD Case Rep.* 2018;4(5):480-481, Figure 1.)

KEY POINTS

- Erythema chronicum migrans classically presents with a bull's eye or targetoid appearance consisting of patches and/or plaques.

- In darker skin, the erythema can appear dusky and violaceous with pallor, particularly at the periphery. In cases where the central bull's eye is less prominent, the condition could be mistaken for urticaria.

- In lighter skin, the concentric rings tend to be bright pink to red.

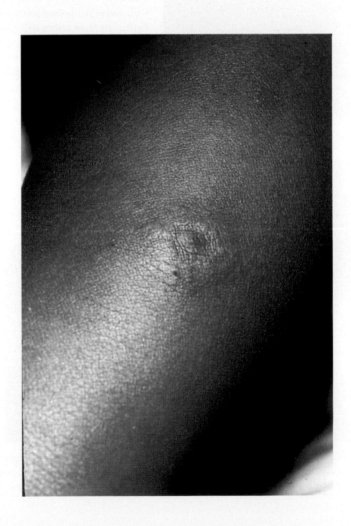

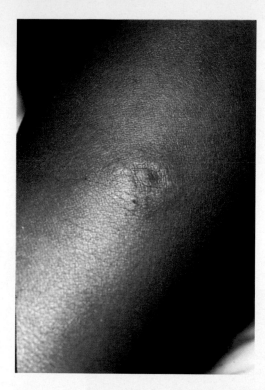

FIGURE 18-1. Targetoid plaque with darker red-brown center and hyperpigmented brown to pink periphery on the lower leg, representing expanding erythema migrans in a patient with darker skin. (Reproduced with permission from Bhate C, Schwartz RA. Lyme disease: Part I. Advances and perspectives. *J Am Acad Dermatol.* 2011;64(4):619-636.)

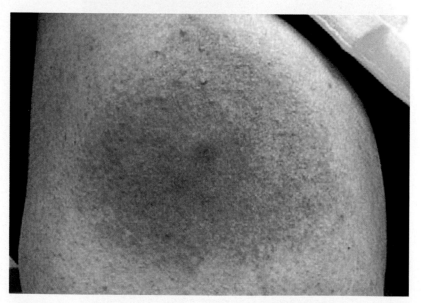

FIGURE 18-2. Large targetoid patch with a central ring of dusky erythema and a lighter pink periphery representing erythema migrans in an individual with light skin. (Reproduced with permission from Bhate C, Schwartz RA. Lyme disease: Part I. Advances and perspectives. *J Am Acad Dermatol.* 2011;64(4):619-636.)

Follicular Disorders

KEY POINTS

- Comedonal, inflammatory, and nodulocystic acne occur in all skin types.

- In darker skin, comedones and inflammatory papules may be skin colored and lack erythema in contrast to lighter skin where they can be skin colored or pink with significant erythema.

- The sequalae of acne can vary significantly across skin colors with postinflammatory pigment alteration occurring in darker skin.

- Atrophic, hypertrophic, and keloidal scarring may also occur in those who are prone, and the latter is more common in skin of color.

- Certain types of acne including pomade acne and steroid-induced acne may occur more commonly in skin of color.

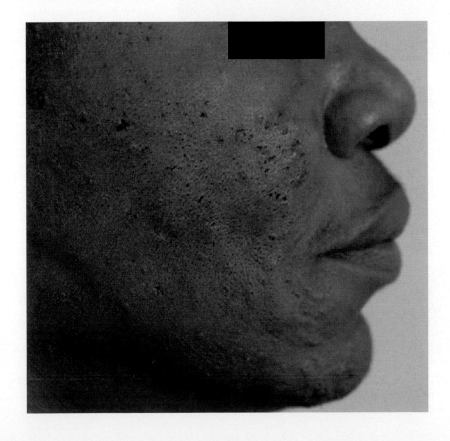

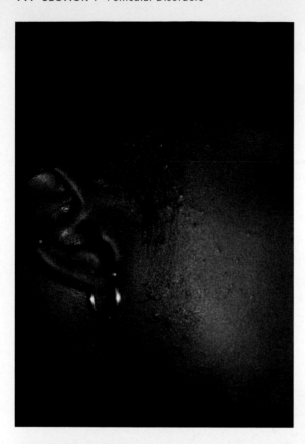

FIGURE 19-1. Skin-colored closed comedones along the temple and lateral cheek secondary to hair oil use and consistent with pomade acne in a dark-skinned person. (Reproduced with permission from Taylor SC, Kelly AP, Lim HW, et al. *Taylor and Kelly's Dermatology for Skin of Color*, 2nd ed. New York, NY: McGraw Hill; 2016, Figure 42-5.)

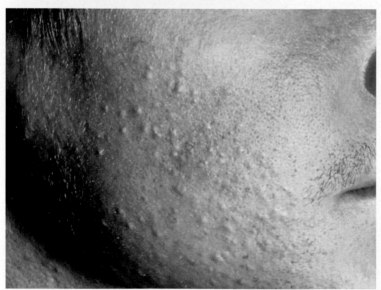

FIGURE 19-2. Open and primarily closed skin-colored comedones along the lateral cheek and jawline. (Reproduced with permission from Baumann L, Saghari S, Weisberg E. *Cosmetic Dermatology: Principles and Practice*, 2nd ed. New York, NY: McGraw Hill; 2009, Figure 12-2.)

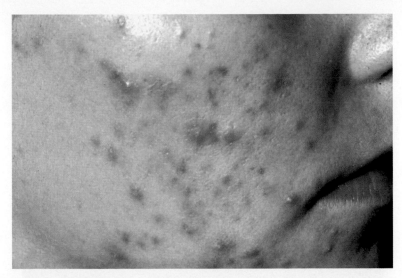

FIGURE 19-3. Pink inflammatory papules and white pustules on the cheek surrounded by pink-brown macules signifying postinflammatory erythema, which is more easily visible in lighter skin. (Reproduced with permission from Baumann L, Saghari S, Weisberg E. *Cosmetic Dermatology: Principles and Practice*, 2nd ed. New York, NY: McGraw Hill; 2009, Figure 12-1.)

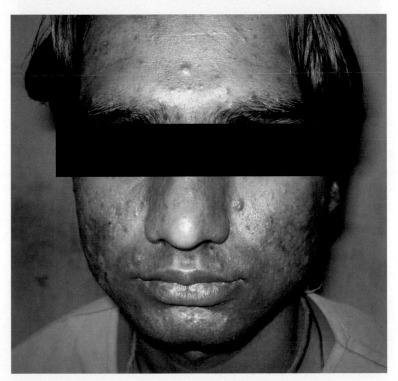

FIGURE 19-4. Pink inflammatory papules scattered diffusely on the face, with background atrophic scarring and brown macules consistent with postinflammatory hyperpigmentation. (Reproduced with permission from Taylor SC, Kelly AP, Lim HW, et al. *Taylor and Kelly's Dermatology for Skin of Color*, 2nd ed. New York, NY: McGraw Hill; 2016, Figure 91-11.)

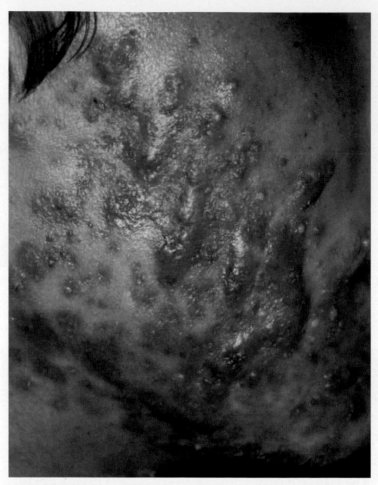

FIGURE 19-5. Bright-pink to red inflammatory papules, nodules, comedones, pustules, and cysts, with surrounding background scarring and pink macules signifying postinflammatory erythema. (Reproduced with permission from Wolff K, Johnson RA, Saavedra AP, et al. *Fitzpatrick's Color Atlas and Synopsis of Clinical Dermatology*, 8th ed. New York, NY: McGraw Hill; 2017, Figure 1-5.)

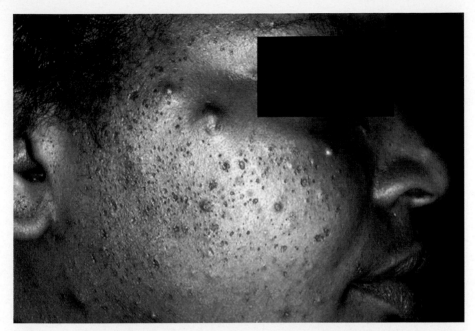

FIGURE 19-6. Brown to violaceous papules and nodules along with comedones and pustules and areas of background erythema most visible along the mid-inferior border of the photo. The patient also has background icepick scarring and violaceous to brown macules signifying postinflammatory pigmentation and chronic acne changes. (Reproduced with permission from Taylor SC, Kelly AP, Lim HW, et al. *Taylor and Kelly's Dermatology for Skin of Color*, 2nd ed. New York, NY: McGraw Hill; 2016, Figure 42-3.)

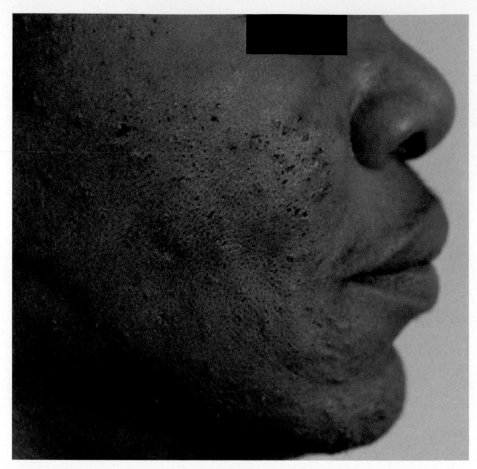

FIGURE 19-7. Skin-colored to dark-brown papules along the cheek, jawline, and chin surrounded by a background of atrophic icepick scarring and brown macules signifying postinflammatory hyperpigmentation. This is an example of a person with new, active acne as well as older acne scarring. (Reproduced with permission from Taylor SC, Kelly AP, Lim HW, et al. *Taylor and Kelly's Dermatology for Skin of Color*, 2nd ed. New York, NY: McGraw Hill; 2016, Figure 6-3.)

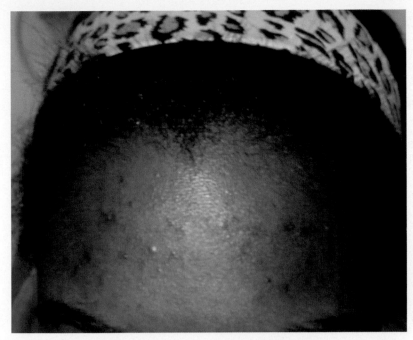

FIGURE 19-8. Pomade acne on the forehead presenting with comedonal acne and background postinflammatory hyperpigmentation. (Reproduced with permission from Taylor SC, Kelly AP, Lim HW, et al. *Taylor and Kelly's Dermatology for Skin of Color*, 2nd ed. New York, NY: McGraw Hill; 2016, Figure 84-3.)

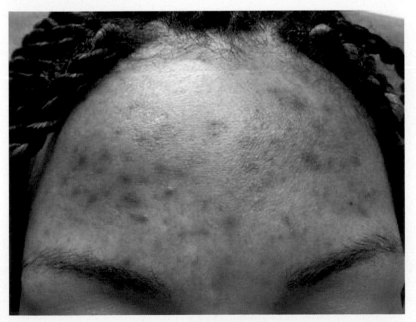

FIGURE 19-9. Dark-brown macules scattered on the forehead along with several closed comedones in a Black woman. (Reproduced with permission from Jackson-Richards D, Pandya AG. *Dermatology Atlas for Skin of Color*. Berlin Heidelberg: Springer-Verlag; 2014.)

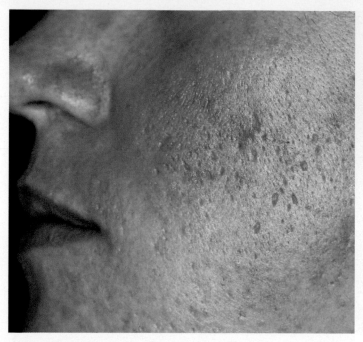

FIGURE 19-10. Icepick atrophic scarring secondary to acne on the cheek of a young woman. (Reproduced with permission from Habif TP. *Clinical Dermatology: A Color Guide to Diagnosis and Therapy*, 5th ed. St. Louis, MO: Elsevier; 2010, Figure 7-44.)

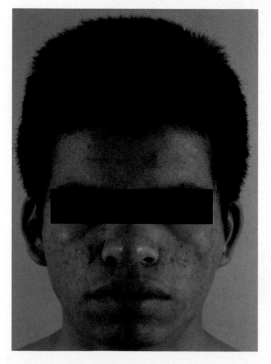

FIGURE 19-11. Atrophic boxcar and icepick scars along the basolateral cheeks with scattered light-brown macules, all of which signify skin changes from resolved acne in a Latino man. (Reproduced with permission from Taylor SC, Kelly AP, Lim HW, et al. *Taylor and Kelly's Dermatology for Skin of Color*, 2nd ed. New York, NY: McGraw Hill; 2016, Figure 42-2.)

KEY POINTS

- The types of cutaneous rosacea include papulopustular, erythematotelangectatic, phymatous, and granulomatous rosacea.

- The papulopustular subtype and granulomatous variant are reported as more common in skin of color.

- This condition is often underdiagnosed and undertreated in skin of color due to increased melanin often masking the erythema and flushing seen with rosacea.

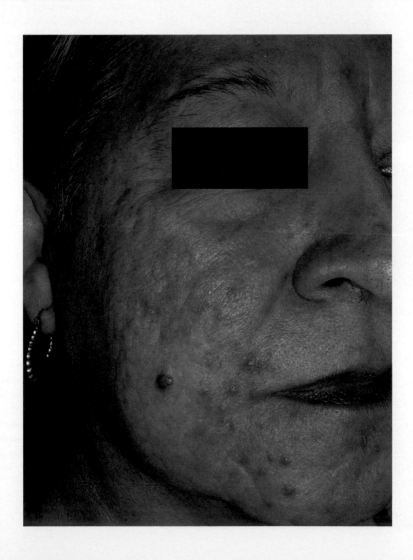

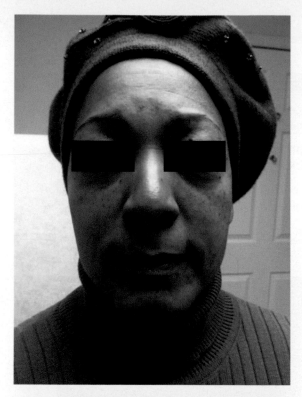

FIGURE 20-1. Background erythema with overlying papules on the medial cheeks, glabella, and chin in a Black woman with rosacea. (Reproduced with permission from Alexis AF, Callender VD, Baldwin HE, et al. Global epidemiology and clinical spectrum of rosacea, highlighting skin of color: Review and clinical practice experience. *J Am Acad Dermatol.* 2019;80(6):1722-1729.)

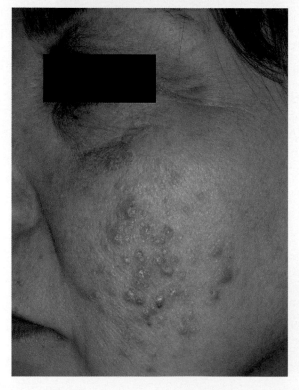

FIGURE 20-2. Bright-pink papules overlying a background of erythema along the nose, cheeks, chin, jawline, and perioral skin. Note the bright-pink telangiectasias along the nasal ala. (From Usatine RP, Smith MA, Mayeaux EJ Jr, et al. *The Color Atlas and Synopsis of Family Medicine,* 3rd ed. New York, NY: McGraw Hill; 2019, Figure 119-8. Reproduced with permission from Richard P. Usatine, MD.)

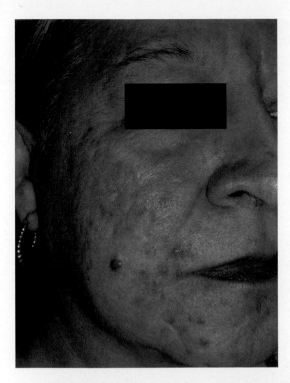

FIGURE 20-3. Pink papules with a background of erythema visible along the right cheek and chin. (From Usatine RP, Smith MA, Mayeaux EJ Jr, et al. *The Color Atlas and Synopsis of Family Medicine*, 3rd ed. New York, NY: McGraw Hill; 2019, Figure 119-9. Reproduced with permission from Richard P. Usatine, MD.)

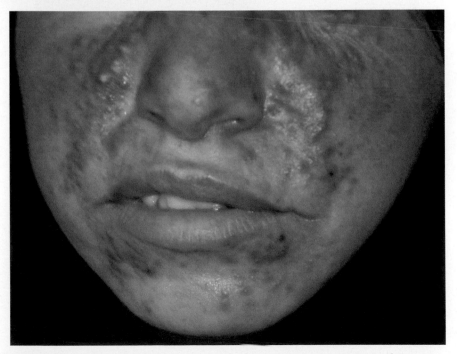

FIGURE 20-4. Inflammatory papules and pustules on the cheek and perioral skin of a young Middle Eastern woman. (Reproduced with permission from Taylor SC, Kelly AP, Lim HW, et al. *Taylor and Kelly's Dermatology for Skin of Color*, 2nd ed. New York, NY: McGraw Hill; 2016, Figure 92-8.)

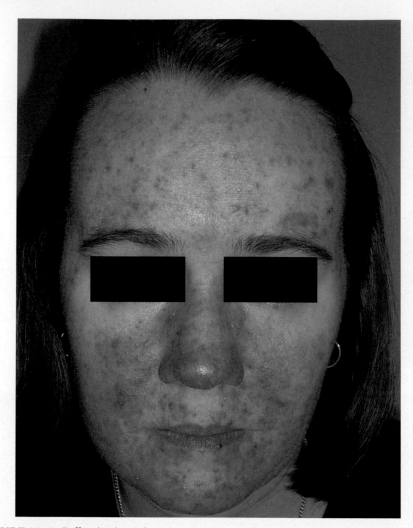

FIGURE 20-5. Diffuse bright-pink–red erythema on the face, with periocular sparing and overlying inflammatory papules. (From Usatine RP, Smith MA, Mayeaux EJ Jr, et al. *The Color Atlas and Synopsis of Family Medicine*, 3rd ed. New York, NY: McGraw Hill; 2019, Figure 119-1. Reproduced with permission from Richard P. Usatine, MD.)

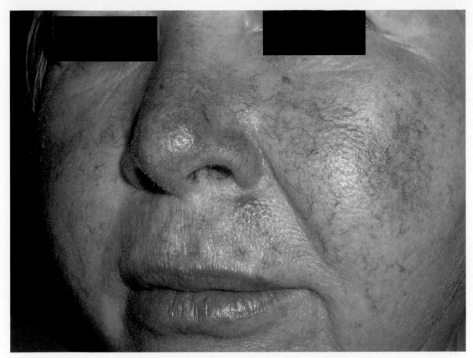

FIGURE 20-6. Bright-pink telangiectatic patches along the nose, cheeks, and upper cutaneous lip, with an inflammatory papule visible inferior to the left nasal ala in a middle-aged Hispanic woman. (From Usatine RP, Smith MA, Mayeaux EJ Jr, et al. *The Color Atlas and Synopsis of Family Medicine*, 3rd ed. New York, NY: McGraw Hill; 2019, Figure 119-6. Reproduced with permission from Richard P. Usatine, MD.)

KEY POINTS

- Perioral dermatitis can involve the cheeks, nasolabial folds, and chin in all skin types.

- It can occur secondary to long-term topical steroid use, which can be found in many skin-lightening products used in populations with skin of color.

- Clinically it can present with pink to skin-colored papules on lighter skin with intense background erythema. In contrast, darker skin tends to present with skin-colored to pink-brown papules with less visible background erythema and pigmentation.

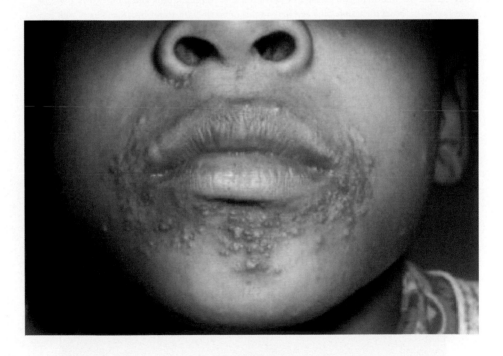

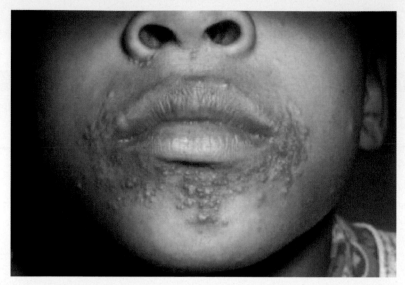

FIGURE 21-1. Periorally and perinasally clustered and confluent pink and pink-brown papules of varying sizes. Note the visible pink erythema inferior to the mid-lower lip. (Reproduced with permission from Prose NS, Kristal L. *Weinberg's Color Atlas of Pediatric Dermatology*, 5th ed. New York, NY: McGraw Hill; 2017, Figure 2-40.)

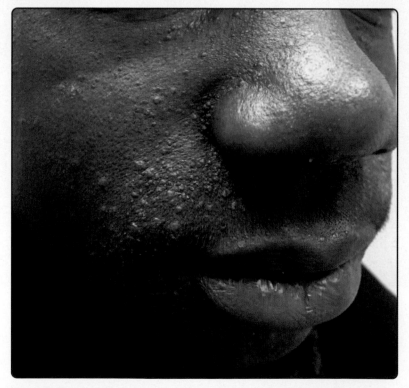

FIGURE 21-2. Perioral pink and light-brown papules of varying sizes extending up to the cheek and infraorbital skin. (Reproduced with permission from Kang S, Amagai M, Bruckner AL, et al. *Fitzpatrick's Dermatology*, 9th ed. New York, NY: McGraw Hill; 2019, Figure 80-6.)

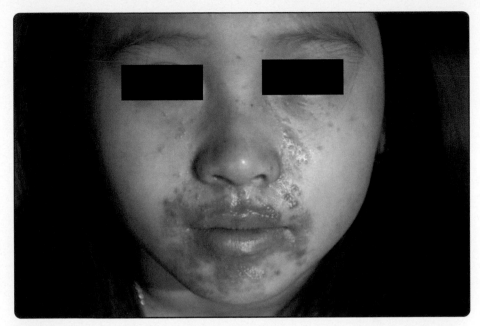

FIGURE 21-3. Pink confluent papules and plaques on the medial cheeks and periorally in a young Asian woman. (Reproduced with permission from Kang S, Amagai M, Bruckner AL, et al. *Fitzpatrick's Dermatology*, 9th ed. New York, NY: McGraw Hill; 2019, Figure 104-6.)

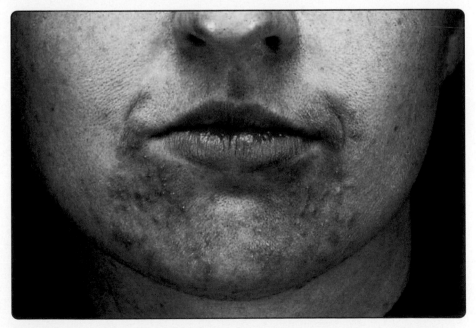

FIGURE 21-4. Bright-red papules overlying an erythematous patch lateral to the commissures and on the chin. (Reproduced with permission from Desman GT, Barnhill RL. *Barnhill's Dermatopathology Challenge: Self-Assessment & Review*. New York, NY: McGraw Hill; 2016, Chapter 2.)

KEY POINTS

- Folliculitis can occur anywhere on the body secondary to various infectious etiologies.

- It can present with various papular morphologies including flat topped, pinpoint, umbilciated, and nodular.

- Clinically on lighter skin it presents with pink to red papules while on darker skin these papules can be pink to pink brown to violaceous to dark brown. Both skin types can also present with pustules.

- In darker skin, it can also resolve with postinflamammatory hyperpigmentation.

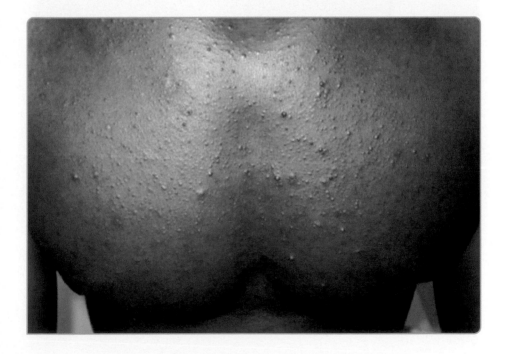

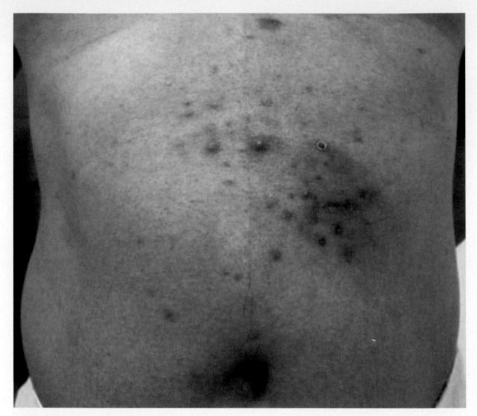

FIGURE 22-1. Perifollicular pink papules surrounded by brown macules signifying postinflammatory hyperpigmentation on the abdomen of a Hispanic man. Note on the left mid-abdomen the brown papules with surrounding brown pigmentation signifying resolving inflammatory papules with background postinflammatory changes. (From Taylor SC, Kelly AP, Lim HW, et al. *Taylor and Kelly's Dermatology for Skin of Color*, 2nd ed. New York, NY: McGraw Hill; 2016, Figure 41-1B. Reproduced with permission from the Ronald O. Perelman Department of Dermatology, New York University School of Medicine, NYU Langone Medical Center, New York.)

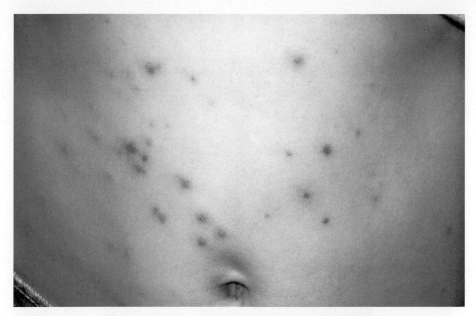

FIGURE 22-2. Distinct bright-pink perifollicular papules on the abdomen. Note the lack of background pigmentary change. (Reproduced with permission from Prose NS, Kristal L. *Weinberg's Color Atlas of Pediatric Dermatology*, 5th ed. New York, NY: McGraw Hill; 2017, Figure 3-16.)

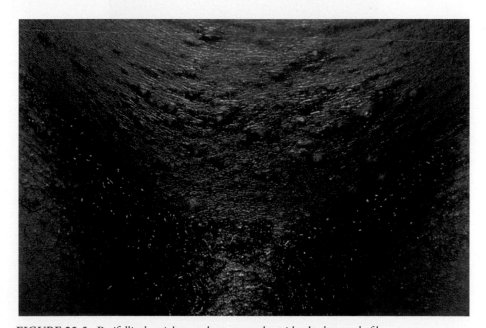

FIGURE 22-3. Perifollicular violaceous brown papules with a background of brown hyperpigmentation on the suprapubic region of a Black male. Note the more visible erythema of the excoriated papule located superiorly. (Reproduced with permission from Taylor SC, Kelly AP, Lim HW, et al. *Taylor and Kelly's Dermatology for Skin of Color*, 2nd ed. New York, NY: McGraw Hill; 2016, Figure 39-2.)

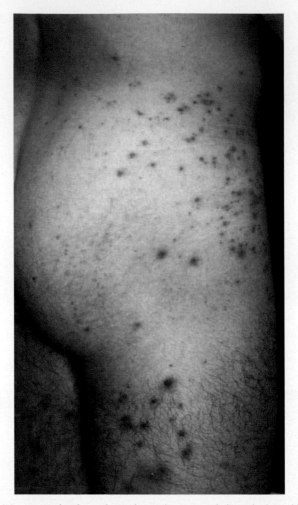

FIGURE 22-4. Magenta and red papules and macules scattered along the lateral buttock and posterior thigh from an infectious folliculitis. (Reproduced with permission from Wolff K, Johnson RA, Saavedra AP, et al. *Fitzpatrick's Color Atlas and Synopsis of Clinical Dermatology*, 8th ed. New York, NY: McGraw Hill; 2017, Figure 25-18.)

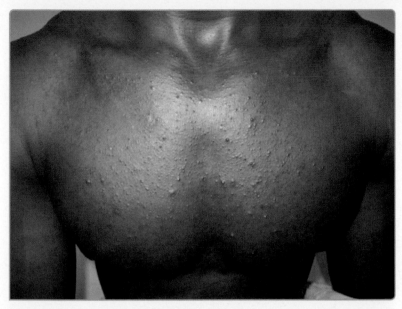

FIGURE 22-5. Scattered skin-colored papules and pustules on the anterior chest of a dark-skinned person who has ill-defined background brown pigmentary change. (Reproduced with permission from Kang S, Amagai M, Bruckner AL, et al. *Fitzpatrick's Dermatology*, 9th ed. New York, NY: McGraw Hill; 2019, Figure 161-13A.)

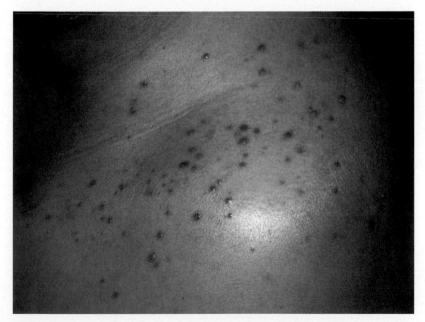

FIGURE 22-6. Distinct, scattered violaceous papules along the shoulder of a dark-skinned person, signifying early, active folliculitis prior to the onset of any postinflammatory pigment changes. (From Usatine RP, Smith MA, Mayeaux EJ Jr, et al. *The Color Atlas and Synopsis of Family Medicine*, 3rd ed. New York, NY: McGraw Hill; 2019, Figure 123-3. Reproduced with permission from Richard P. Usatine, MD.)

KEY POINTS

- Hidradenitis suppurativa is a chronic inflammatory disease consisting of recurrent nodules, plaques, sinus tracts, fistulas, and scarring in intertriginous areas.

- In lighter skin, this can be seen as pink to red in color in contrast to the violaceous or brawny appearance in skin of color.

- In darker skin, later stages of the disease can present with hypertrophic or keloidal scarring.

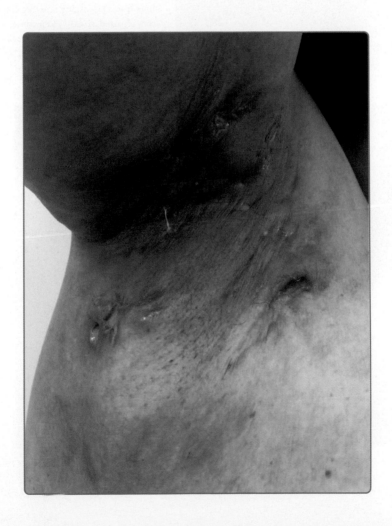

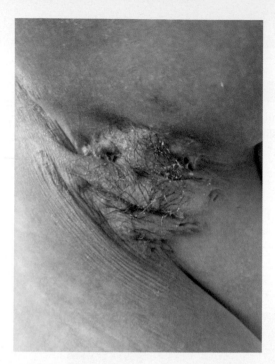

FIGURE 23-1. Purple-brown atrophic scars with surrounding linear cords and sinus tracts signifying scarring changes from chronic disease. (Reproduced with permission from Burgin S. *Guidebook to Dermatologic Diagnosis.* New York, NY: McGraw Hill; 2021, Figure 12-19.)

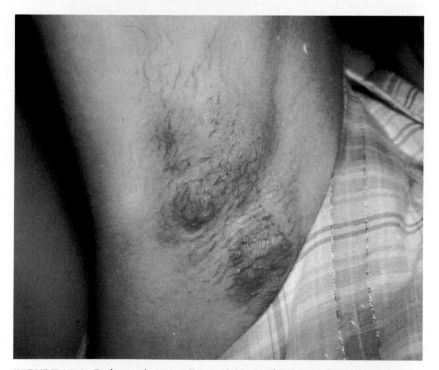

FIGURE 23-2. Pink protuberant axillary nodules signifying active disease without sinus tracts or scarring that can be seen with more chronic disease. (Reproduced with permission from Prose NS, Kristal L. *Weinberg's Color Atlas of Pediatric Dermatology,* 5th ed. New York, NY: McGraw Hill; 2017, Figure 2-34.)

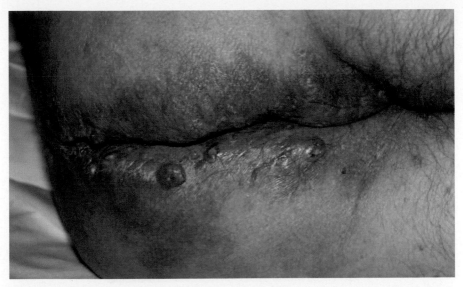

FIGURE 23-3. Pink to pink-brown nodules with background brawny erythema along the gluteal cleft. (Reproduced with permission from Taylor SC, Kelly AP, Lim HW, et al. *Taylor and Kelly's Dermatology for Skin of Color*, 2nd ed. New York, NY: McGraw Hill; 2016, Figure 43-2B.)

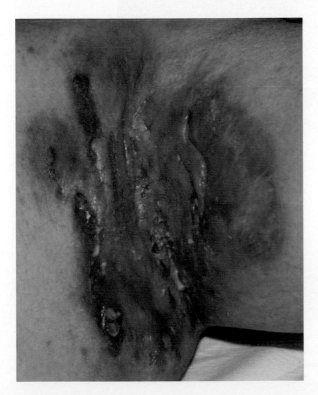

FIGURE 23-4. Pink to brown confluent patches, plaques, nodules, and linear cords with areas of overlying ulcerations and pustular drainage in the right axilla signifying active Hurley stage III disease. (Reproduced with permission from Taylor SC, Kelly AP, Lim HW, et al. *Taylor and Kelly's Dermatology for Skin of Color*, 2nd ed. New York, NY: McGraw Hill; 2016, Figure 43-1B.)

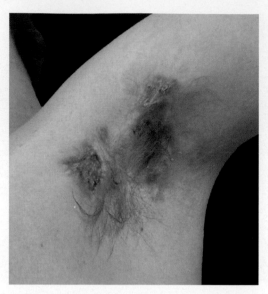

FIGURE 23-5. Pink atrophic plaques with surrounding linear cords and pink and brown patches signifying postinflammatory pigmentary changes from chronic disease in a young man. (Reproduced with permission from Wolff K, Johnson RA, Saavedra AP, et al. *Fitzpatrick's Color Atlas and Synopsis of Clinical Dermatology*, 8th ed. New York, NY: McGraw Hill; 2017, Figure 1-18.)

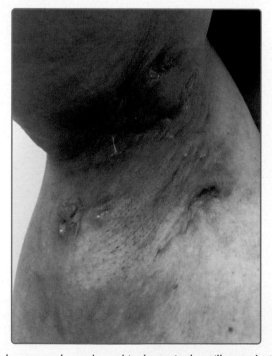

FIGURE 23-6. Violaceous patches and atrophic plaques in the axillary vault signifying chronic diseases with several active pink ulcerations at the inferior border of the axilla. (Reproduced with permission from Kang S, Amagai M, Bruckner AL, et al. *Fitzpatrick's Dermatology*, 9th ed. New York, NY: McGraw Hill; 2019, Figure 84-4.)

KEY POINTS

- Pseudofolliculitis barbae is a chronic follicular disorder more commonly seen in men and hirsute women of color.

- In the mild stage, it can present as perifollicular papules. In lighter skin, it can be pink to red, while in darker skin, it can range from skin colored to pink-brown or dark brown.

- Chronic disease can include keloids, hypertrophic and atrophic scarring, and postinflammatory pigment alteration.

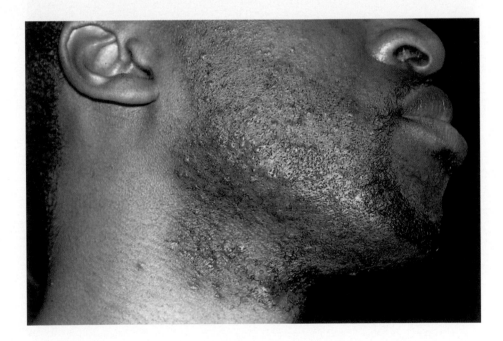

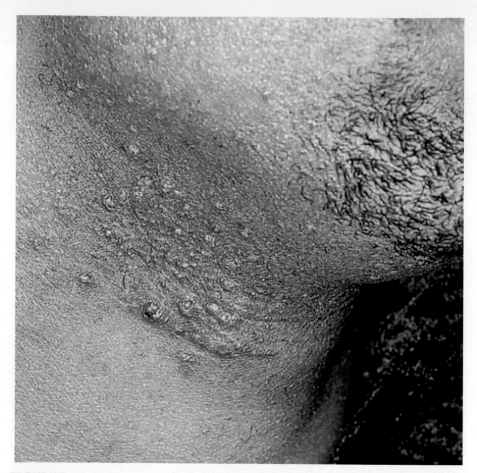

FIGURE 24-1. Pink to pink-brown perifollicular papules with background hyperpigmentation along the anterior neck. Note the lack of inflammation in the areas of longer hair on the chin. (Reproduced with permission from Wolff K, Johnson RA, Saavedra AP, et al. *Fitzpatrick's Color Atlas and Synopsis of Clinical Dermatology*, 8th ed. New York, NY: McGraw Hill; 2017, Figure 31-22.)

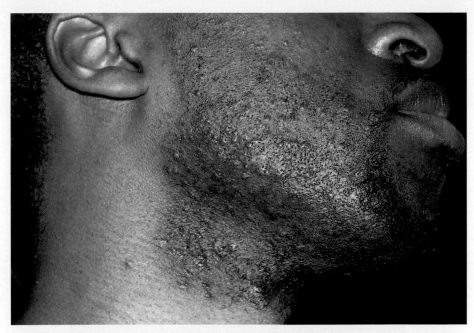

FIGURE 24-2. Skin-colored to dark-brown perifollicular papules densely scattered along the hair-bearing areas of the face in a young Black man. Note the diffuse background of hyperpigmentation from chronic inflammation, which is sharply demarcated from normal skin along the lateral neck and cheek. Also note the lack of these changes in areas with longer hair periorally. (Reproduced with permission from Kang S, Amagai M, Bruckner AL, et al. *Fitzpatrick's Dermatology*, 9th ed. New York, NY: McGraw Hill; 2019, Figure 150-7.)

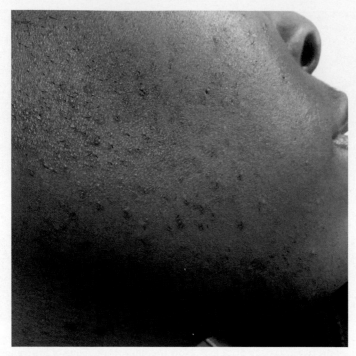

FIGURE 24-3. Dark-brown hyperpigmented macules and fine papules signifying postinflammatory pigmentary changes form pseudofolliculitis barbae in a Black woman. (Reproduced with permission from Kang S, Amagai M, Bruckner AL, et al. *Fitzpatrick's Dermatology*, 9th ed. New York, NY: McGraw Hill; 2019, Figure 90-4.)

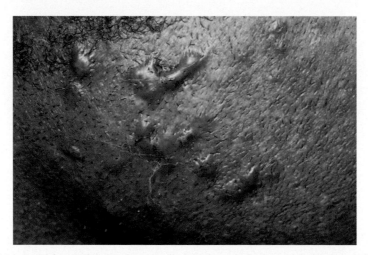

FIGURE 24-4. Pink to pink-brown hypertrophic keloids on the jawline induced by pseudofolliculitis barbae. (Reproduced with permission from Taylor SC, Kelly AP, Lim HW, et al. *Taylor and Kelly's Dermatology for Skin of Color*, 2nd ed. New York, NY: McGraw Hill; 2016, Figure 39-5.)

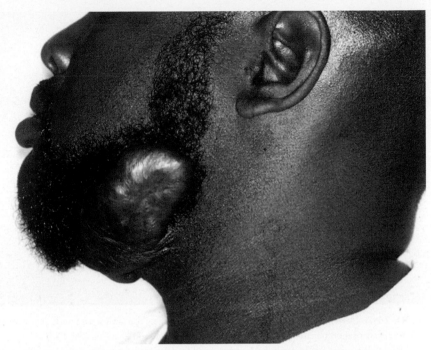

FIGURE 24-5. Skin colored large keloid along the jawline secondary to pseudofolliculitis barbae. (Reproduced with permission from Taylor SC, Kelly AP, Lim HW, et al. *Taylor and Kelly's Dermatology for Skin of Color*, 2nd ed. New York, NY: McGraw Hill; 2016, Figure 39-6.)

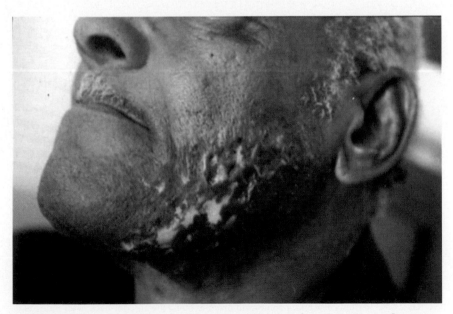

FIGURE 24-6. Dark brown hyerprtrophic scarring with areas of atrophy and postinflammatory hypopigmentation signifying a range chronic changes from pseudfolliculitis barbae. (Reproduced with permission from Taylor SC, Kelly AP, Lim HW, et al. *Taylor and Kelly's Dermatology for Skin of Color*, 2nd ed. New York, NY: McGraw Hill; 2016, Figure 39-7.)

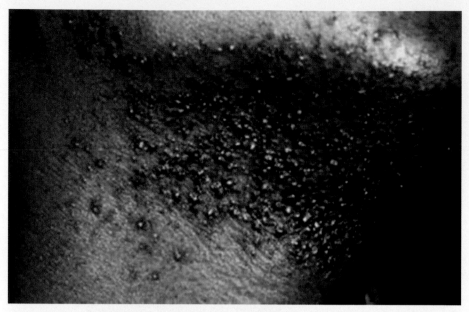

FIGURE 24-7. Dense proliferation of dark brown papules along the jawline and neck demonstrating active and severe pseudofolliculitis barbae. (Reproduced with permission from Gray J, McMichael AJ. Pseudofolliculitis barbae: Understanding the condition and the role of facial grooming. *Int J Cosmet Sci.* 2016;38(Suppl 1):24-27.)

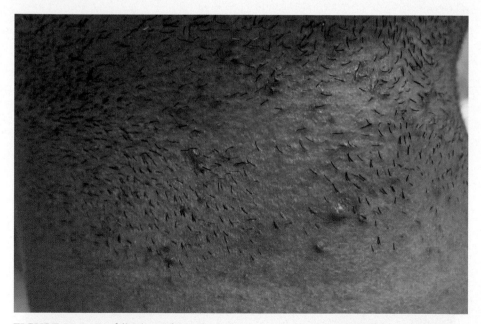

FIGURE 24-8. Perifollicular pink papules and macules along the anterior neck in an individual with lighter skin. (Reproduced with permission from Burgin S: *Guidebook to Dermatologic Diagnosis.* New York, NY: McGraw Hill; 2021, Figure 2-17.)

KEY POINTS

- Acne keloidalis nuchae is a chronic folliculitis on the occipital neck that tends to predominantly affect men of color with coarse, curly hair.

- In early stages, it can present with papules of variable size and color ranging from pink to pink-brown in lighter skin and brown to dark brown in darker skin. Pustules may be observed in more active disease.

- In late stages, it can present with numerous and large keloidal plaques and postinflammatory pigmentation alteration.

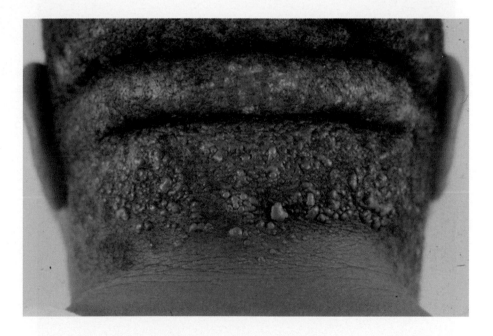

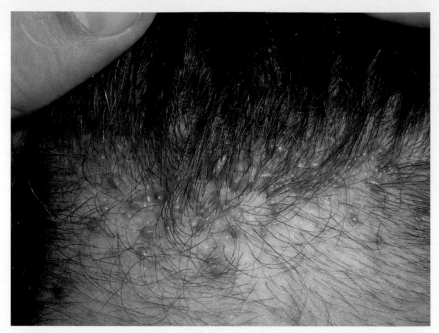

FIGURE 25-1. Perifollicular clustered pink papules and pustules on the neck of a young Hispanic man. (From Usatine RP, Smith MA, Mayeaux EJ Jr, et al. *The Color Atlas and Synopsis of Family Medicine,* 3rd ed. New York, NY: McGraw Hill; 2019, Figure 123-5. Reproduced with permission from Richard P. Usatine, MD.)

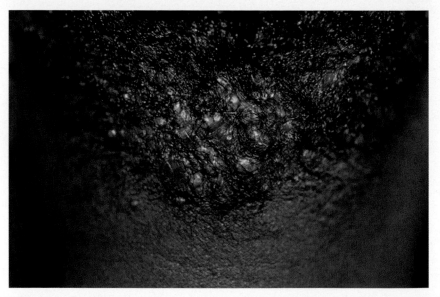

FIGURE 25-2. Perifollicular pink-brown and skin-colored papules clustered on the occipital scalp, signifying earlier stage disease. (Reproduced with permission from Taylor SC, Kelly AP, Lim HW, et al. *Taylor and Kelly's Dermatology for Skin of Color,* 2nd ed. New York, NY: McGraw Hill; 2016, Figure 34-2.)

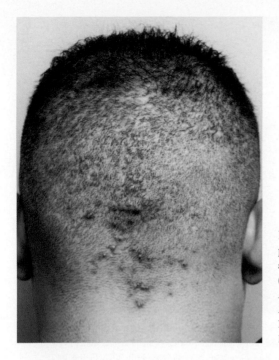

FIGURE 25-3. Small, pink, clustered perifollicular papules on the occipital scalp of a light-skinned person. (Reproduced with permission from Ali A. *McGraw-Hill Education Specialty Board Review Dermatology: A Pictorial Review*, 3rd ed. New York, NY: McGraw Hill; 2015, Figure 1-19.)

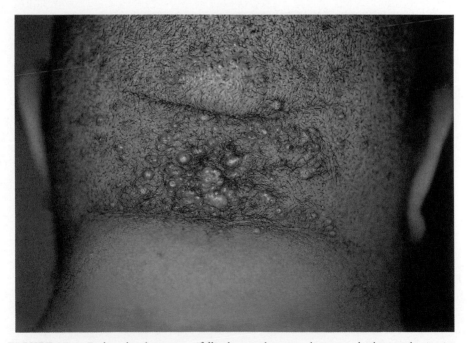

FIGURE 25-4. Pink and violaceous perifollicular papules, some distinct and others coalescing into small keloidal plaques on the occipital scalp of a dark-skinned man. (Reproduced with permission from Soutor C, Hordinsky MK. *Clinical Dermatology*. New York, NY: McGraw Hill; 2013, Figure 19-14.)

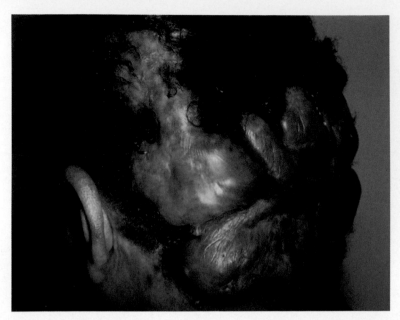

FIGURE 25-5. Large coalescing dark-brown to skin-colored keloids on the occipital scalp secondary to acne keloidalis nuchae. (Reproduced with permission from Taylor SC, Kelly AP, Lim HW, et al. *Taylor and Kelly's Dermatology for Skin of Color*, 2nd ed. New York, NY: McGraw Hill; 2016, Figure 34-7.)

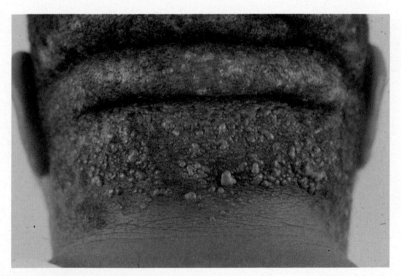

FIGURE 25-6. Numerous skin-colored and pink-brown papules on the occipital scalp in a Black male with active acne keloidalis nuchae. (Reproduced with permission from Taylor SC, Kelly AP, Lim HW, et al. *Taylor and Kelly's Dermatology for Skin of Color*, 2nd ed. New York, NY: McGraw Hill; 2016, Figure 34-3.)

Benign Neoplasms

SECTION

Benign Neoplasms

KEY POINTS

- Seborrheic keratoses are benign epidermal neoplasms that can occur in any skin color.

- In lighter skin, they are often pink to tan, while in darker skin, they are often brown to black.

- In certain populations of color, seborrheic keratoses are considered a manifestation of photoaging.

- Darker and smaller seborrheic keratoses are called dermatosis papulosis nigra and more commonly present on the face.

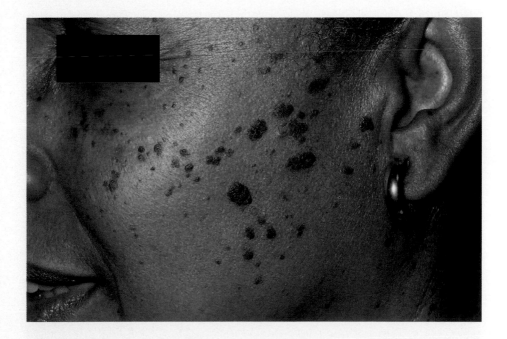

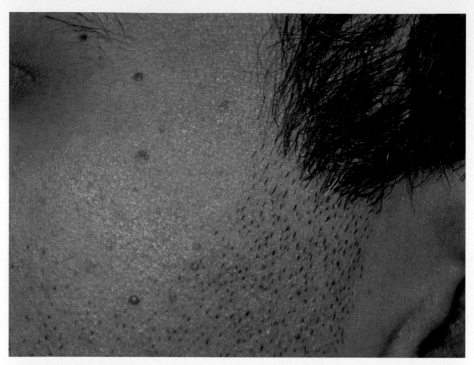

FIGURE 26-1. Small light-brown papules along the lateral face of an Asian man. (Reproduced with permission from Taylor SC, Kelly AP, Lim HW, et al. *Taylor and Kelly's Dermatology for Skin of Color*, 2nd ed. New York, NY: McGraw Hill; 2016, Figure 87-3.)

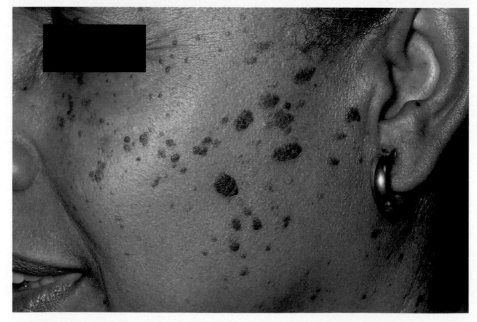

FIGURE 26-2. Small brown to large black flat-topped stuck-on papules along the face and neck of a woman with dark skin. (Reproduced with permission from Wolff K, Johnson RA, Saavedra AP, et al. *Fitzpatrick's Color Atlas and Synopsis of Clinical Dermatology*, 8th ed. New York, NY: McGraw Hill; 2017, Figure 9-37.)

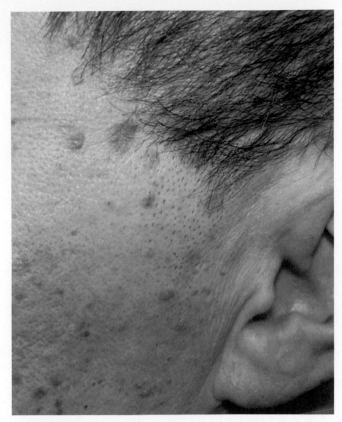

FIGURE 26-3. Tan to light-brown macules and papules scattered along the lateral face of a person with light skin. (Reproduced with permission from Kang S, Amagai M, Bruckner AL, et al. *Fitzpatrick's Dermatology*, 9th ed. New York, NY: McGraw Hill; 2019, Figure 108-4A.)

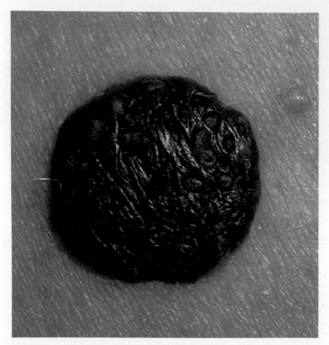

FIGURE 26-4. Discrete dark-brown papule with multiple horn cysts. (From Usatine RP, Smith MA, Mayeaux EJ Jr, et al. *The Color Atlas and Synopsis of Family Medicine*, 3rd ed. New York, NY: McGraw Hill; 2019, Figure 164-4. Reproduced with permission from Richard P. Usatine, MD.)

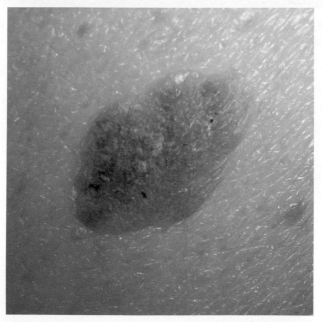

FIGURE 26-5. Discrete tan waxy stuck-on scaly papule. (From Usatine RP, Smith MA, Mayeaux EJ Jr, et al. *The Color Atlas and Synopsis of Family Medicine*, 3rd ed. New York, NY: McGraw Hill; 2019, Figure 164-5. Reproduced with permission from Richard P. Usatine, MD.)

KEY POINTS

- Dermatofibromas are solitary neoplasms that can vary in morphology and color.

- The morphology across skin types can be flat or nodular and exophytic.

- Dermatofibroma sarcoma protuberans is a tissue sarcoma that tends to present as keloidal-appearing nodules coalescing into plaques.

- For both conditions, in lighter skin, it is often pink to skin colored, while in darker skin, it can be violaceous to pink-brown or gray-brown.

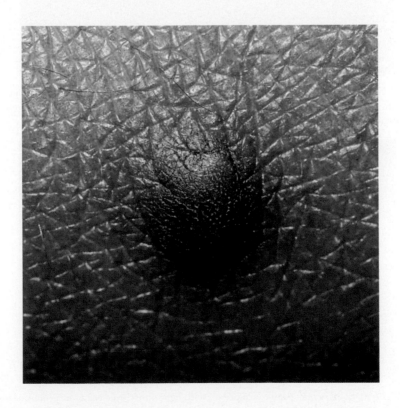

DERMATOFIBROMA

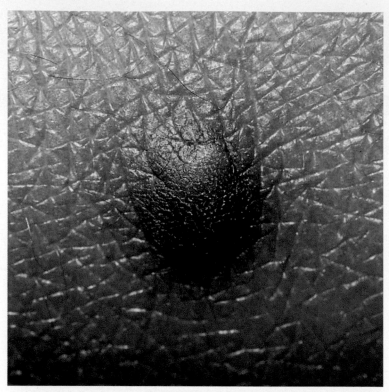

FIGURE 27-1. Solitary dark-brown to black papule on a person with dark skin. (Reproduced with permission from Wolff K, Johnson RA, Saavedra AP, et al. *Fitzpatrick's Color Atlas and Synopsis of Clinical Dermatology*, 8th ed. New York, NY: McGraw Hill; 2017, Figure 9-48B.)

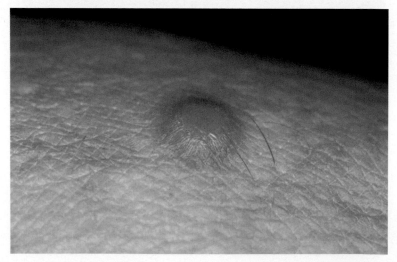

FIGURE 27-2. Solitary pink papule on a person with light skin. (Reproduced with permission from Wolff K, Johnson RA, Saavedra AP, et al. *Fitzpatrick's Color Atlas and Synopsis of Clinical Dermatology*, 8th ed. New York, NY: McGraw Hill; 2017, Figure 9-48A.)

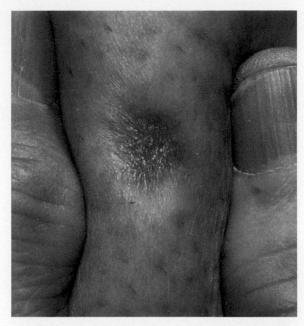

FIGURE 27-3. Bright pink macule showing positive dimple sign on lighter skin. (Reproduced with permission from Wolff K, Johnson RA, Saavedra AP, et al. *Fitzpatrick's Color Atlas and Synopsis of Clinical Dermatology*, 8th ed. New York, NY: McGraw Hill; 2017, Figure 9-48C.)

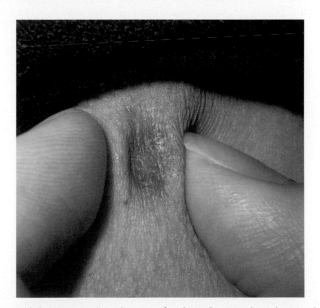

FIGURE 27-4. Pink-brown macule with a rim of pink erythema and overlying scale exhibiting a positive dimple sign. (From Usatine RP, Smith MA, Mayeaux EJ Jr, et al. *The Color Atlas and Synopsis of Family Medicine*, 3rd ed. New York, NY: McGraw Hill; 2019, Figure 166-3. Reproduced with permission from Richard P. Usatine, MD.)

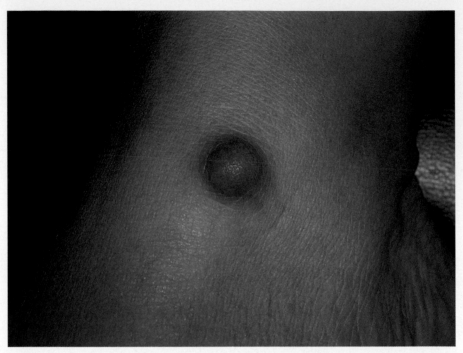

FIGURE 27-5. Solitary brown-gray nodule on a person with dark skin. (From Usatine RP, Smith MA, Mayeaux EJ Jr, et al. *The Color Atlas and Synopsis of Family Medicine*, 3rd ed. New York, NY: McGraw Hill; 2019, Figure 110-9. Reproduced with permission from Richard P. Usatine, MD.)

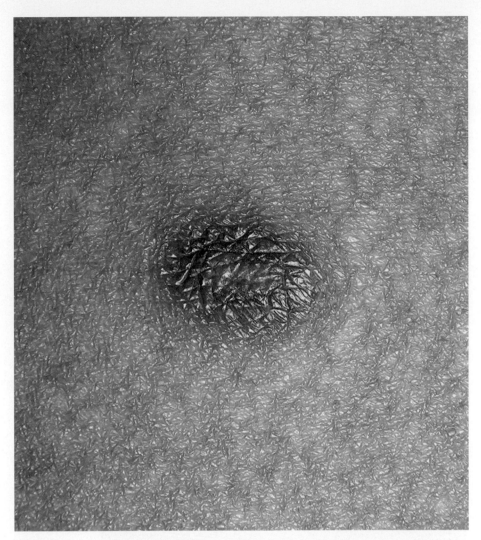

FIGURE 27-6. Dark-brown macule with a rim of pink-brown erythema on a person with dark skin. Typically on palpation, these neoplasms have underlying nodularity and a positive dimple sign. Note the flat presentation, which is in contrast to the dome-shaped morphology that can also occur. (From Usatine RP, Smith MA, Mayeaux EJ Jr, et al. *The Color Atlas and Synopsis of Family Medicine*, 3rd ed. New York, NY: McGraw Hill; 2019, Figure 166-2. Reproduced with permission from Richard P. Usatine, MD.)

DERMATOFIBROMA SARCOMA PROTUBERANS

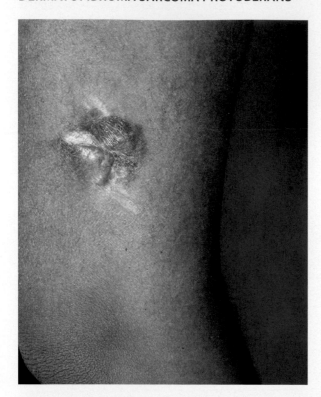

FIGURE 27-7. Pink-brown keloidal plaque with surrounding hyperpigmentation and hypopigmentation on a person with dark skin. (Reproduced with permission from Burgin S. *Guidebook to Dermatologic Diagnosis*, New York, NY: McGraw Hill; 2021, Figure 9-47.)

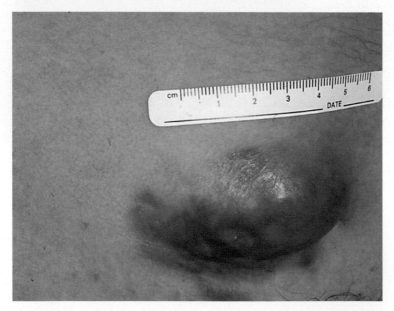

FIGURE 27-8. Pink-brown exophytic tumor with smooth surface on the abdomen of a person with light skin. (Reproduced with permission from Burgin S. *Guidebook to Dermatologic Diagnosis*, New York, NY: McGraw Hill; 2021, Figure 9-43.)

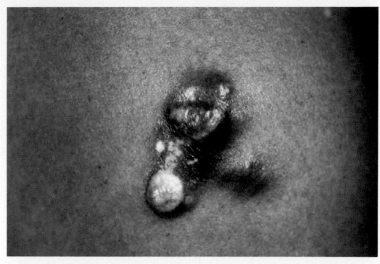

FIGURE 27-9. Multinodular exophytic plaque with shades of white, pink, tan, and brown representing dermatofibrosarcoma protuberans on the trunk of a Black individual. (Reproduced with permission from Gloster HM Jr, Neal K. Skin cancer in skin of color. *J Am Acad Dermatol.* 2006;55(5):741-760.)

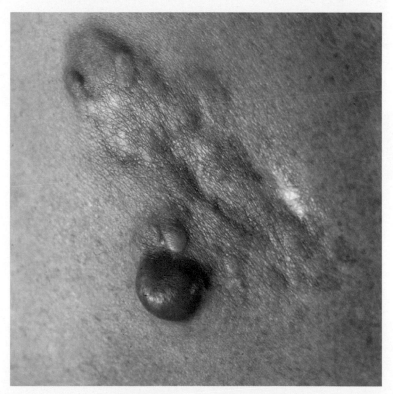

FIGURE 27-10. Pink to red keloidal plaque with protuberant papular component inferiorly in a person with lighter skin. (Reproduced with permission from Wolff K, Johnson RA, Saavedra AP, et al. *Fitzpatrick's Color Atlas and Synopsis of Clinical Dermatology,* 8th ed. New York, NY: McGraw Hill; 2017, Figure 21-22.)

KEY POINTS

- Keloids and hypertrophic scars present as plaques and nodules in areas of prior trauma.

- Keloids are more common in skin of color. They can be very disfiguring, symptomatic, and have profound effects on quality of life.

- Both scar types differ in color, with varying colors of pink to red in lighter skin and skin colored to violaceous or dark brown in darker skin.

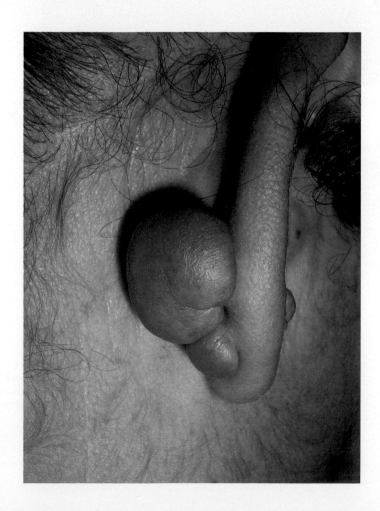

KELOIDS

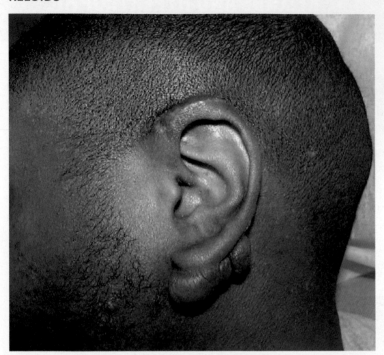

FIGURE 28-1. Skin-colored to dark-brown nodule on the posterior earlobe secondary to piercing. (Reproduced with permission from Avram MR, Avram MM, Ratner D. *Procedural Dermatology*. New York, NY: McGraw Hill; 2015, Figure 23-35.)

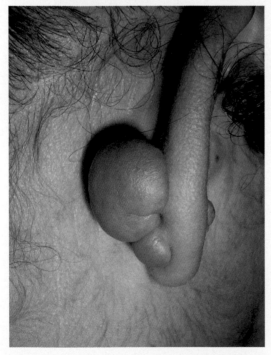

FIGURE 28-2. Pink exophytic nodule on the posterior earlobe secondary to a piercing. (From Usatine RP, Smith MA, Mayeaux EJ Jr, et al. *The Color Atlas and Synopsis of Family Medicine*, 3rd ed. New York, NY: McGraw Hill; 2019, Figure 213-2. Reproduced with permission from Richard P. Usatine, MD.)

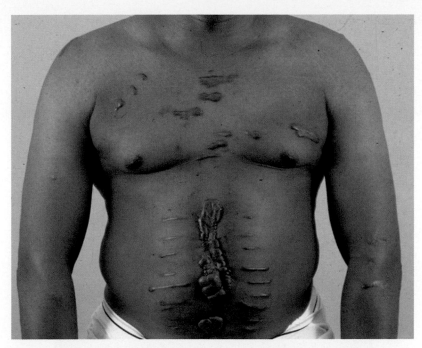

FIGURE 28-3. Dark-brown linear papules and plaques on the anterior trunk of a Black man secondary to abdominal surgery. (Reproduced with permission from Taylor SC, Kelly AP, Lim HW, et al. *Taylor and Kelly's Dermatology for Skin of Color*, 2nd ed. New York, NY: McGraw Hill; 2016, Figure 33-16.)

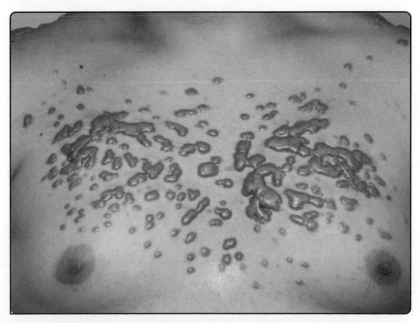

FIGURE 28-4. Pink papules and linear pink plaques on the chest of a person with light skin secondary to acne fulminans. (Reproduced with permission from Kang S, Amagai M, Bruckner AL, et al. *Fitzpatrick's Dermatology*, 9th ed. New York, NY: McGraw Hill; 2019, Figure 80-3D.)

HYPERTROPHIC SCARS

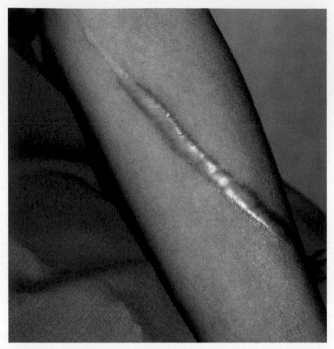

FIGURE 28-5. Pink linear plaque on the upper extremity secondary to a laceration. (Reproduced with permission from Soutor C, Hordinsky MK. *Clinical Dermatology*. New York, NY: McGraw Hill; 2013, Figure 16-9.)

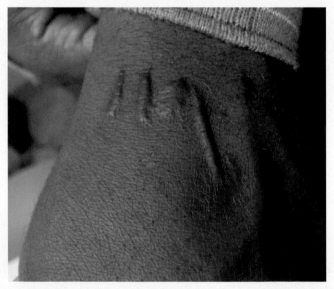

FIGURE 28-6. Multiple linear violaceous plaques on the dorsal hand of a Black person. (Reproduced with permission from Alam M, Bhatia AC, Kundu RV, et al. *Cosmetic Dermatology for Skin of Color*. New York, NY: McGraw Hill; 2009, Figure 13-2.)

Malignancies

KEY POINTS

- While basal cell carcinomas are most commonly seen in those with lighter skin, they can indeed happen in darker skin, and missed and delayed diagnoses can contribute to disease morbidity and even mortality.

- Basal cell carcinomas in darker skin are often pigmented and can mimic melanoma. They can also be mistaken for inflammatory processes.

- The subclassifications of basal cell carcinomas that are seen in lighter skin can also be seen in darker skin. These include superficial, nodular, ulcerative, and morpheaform.

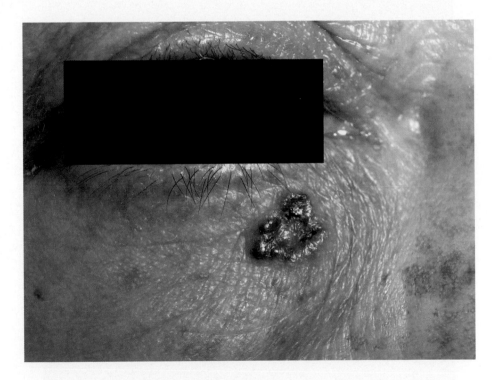

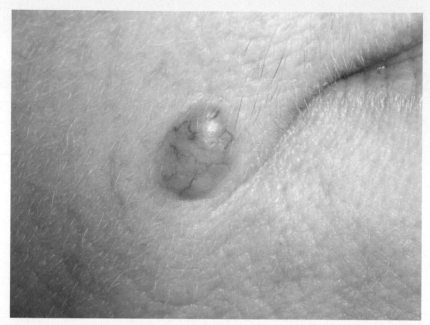

FIGURE 29-1. Well-circumscribed pink pearly telangiectatic papule lateral to the right commissure on the face. (From Usatine RP, Smith MA, Mayeaux EJ Jr, et al. *The Color Atlas and Synopsis of Family Medicine*, 3rd ed. New York, NY: McGraw Hill; 2019, Figure 110-28. Reproduced with permission from Richard P. Usatine, MD.)

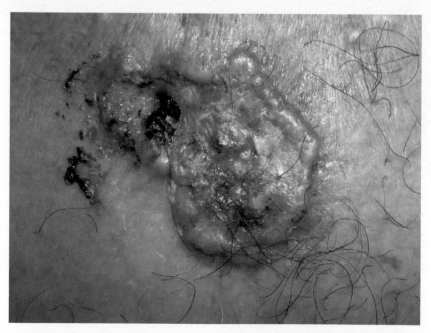

FIGURE 29-2. Close-up of a pink pearly plaque with rolled borders, central ulceration, and overlying hemorrhagic crusting consistent with an ulcerated nodular basal cell carcinoma. (From Usatine RP, Smith MA, Mayeaux EJ Jr, et al. *The Color Atlas and Synopsis of Family Medicine*, 3rd ed. New York, NY: McGraw Hill; 2019, Figure 177-3. Reproduced with permission from Richard P. Usatine, MD.)

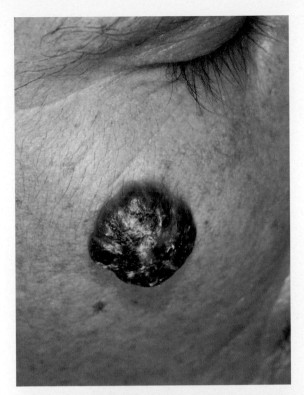

FIGURE 29-3. Well-circumscribed black-gray nodule representing a pigmented basal cell carcinoma on the right cheek, mimicking a nodular melanoma. (From Usatine RP, Smith MA, Mayeaux EJ Jr, et al. *The Color Atlas and Synopsis of Family Medicine*, 3rd ed. New York, NY: McGraw Hill; 2019, Figure 177-11. Reproduced with permission from Richard P. Usatine, MD.)

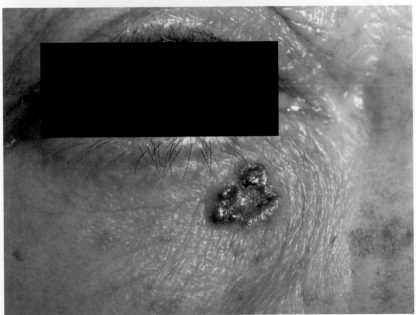

FIGURE 29-4. Well-circumscribed black-gray ulcerated plaque with rolled borders representing a pigmented basal cell carcinoma on the right lower eyelid. (From Usatine RP, Smith MA, Mayeaux EJ Jr, et al. *The Color Atlas and Synopsis of Family Medicine*, 3rd ed. New York, NY: McGraw Hill; 2019, Figure 179-23. Reproduced with permission from Richard P. Usatine, MD.)

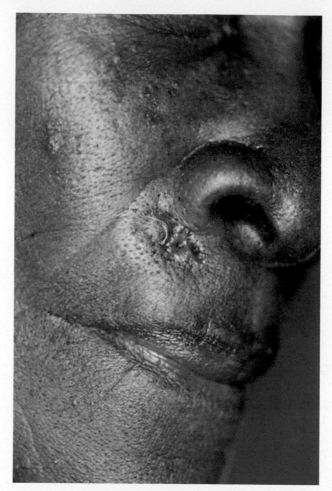

FIGURE 29-5. Atrophic violaceous-pink plaque representing a pigmented basal cell carcinoma on the right upper cutaneous lip of a Black woman. (Reproduced with permission from Taylor SC, Kelly AP, Lim HW, et al. *Taylor and Kelly's Dermatology for Skin of Color*, 2nd ed. New York, NY: McGraw Hill; 2016, Figure 46-2.)

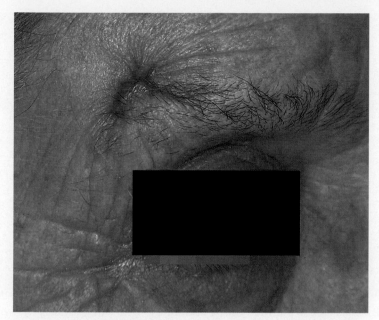

FIGURE 29-6. Atrophic scar-like pink plaque representing a sclerotic basal cell carcinoma on the superior to right lateral eyebrow. (Reproduced with permission from Soutor C, Hordinsky MK. *Clinical Dermatology*. New York, NY: McGraw Hill; 2013, Figure 17-6.)

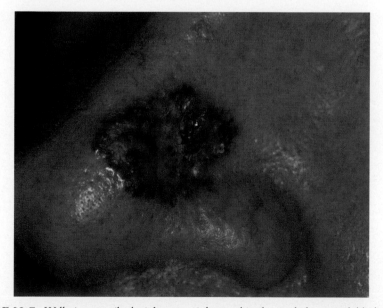

FIGURE 29-7. Well-circumscribed, violaceous-pink, atrophic ulcerated plaque with black finger-like projections along the border and a rim of erythema on the left nose of a Hispanic patient. (Reproduced with permission from Taylor SC, Kelly AP, Lim HW, et al. *Taylor and Kelly's Dermatology for Skin of Color*, 2nd ed. New York, NY: McGraw Hill; 2016, Figure 19-3.)

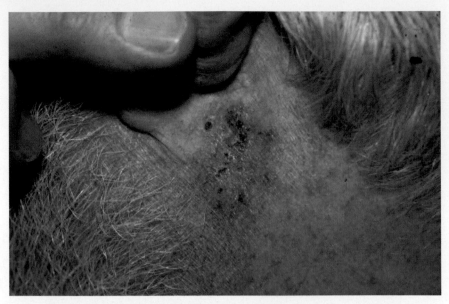

FIGURE 29-8. Pink scaly patch with multiple areas of overlying hemorrhagic crusting representing a superficial basal cell carcinoma on the retroauricular scalp. (Reproduced with permission from Soutor C, Hordinsky MK. *Clinical Dermatology*. New York, NY: McGraw Hill; 2013, Figure 2-32.)

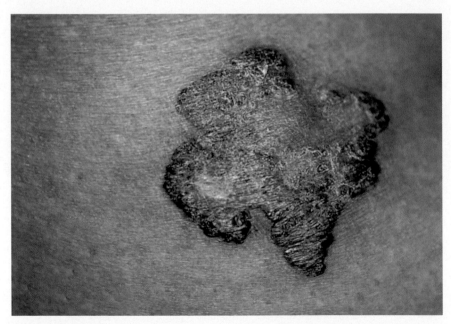

FIGURE 29-9. Dark-brown to black plaque with irregular borders consistent with a pigmented basal cell carcinoma. (Reproduced with permission from Taylor SC, Badreshia S, Callender VD, et al. *Treatments for Skin of Color*. Edinburgh: Saunders Elsevier; 2011, Figure 15.2.)

KEY POINTS

- Squamous cell carcinoma (SCC) is more common in those with lighter skin types; however, it does occur in darker skin and tends to carry greater disease morbidity and mortality in this population.

- In darker skin, it more commonly occurs in an ulcerative form in areas of burns and/or chronic scarring.

- SCCs can mimic the appearance of verruca and basal cell carcinomas.

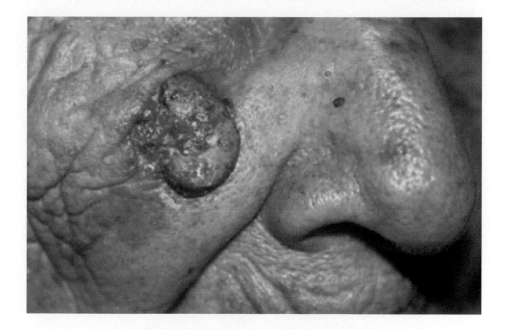

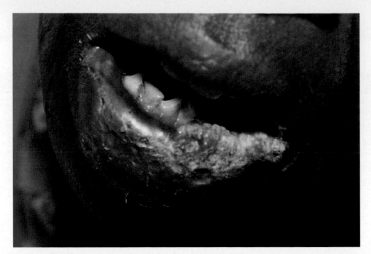

FIGURE 30-1. Pink-white vegetative ulcerated plaque with peripheral crusting representing a Marjolin ulcer arising in a burn on the lower mucocutaneous lip. Note the peripheral hyperpigmentation periorally and on the cheeks from the patient's burn. (From Usatine RP, Smith MA, Mayeaux EJ Jr, et al. *The Color Atlas and Synopsis of Family Medicine*, 3rd ed. New York, NY: McGraw Hill; 2019, Figure 178-3. Reproduced with permission from Richard P. Usatine, MD.)

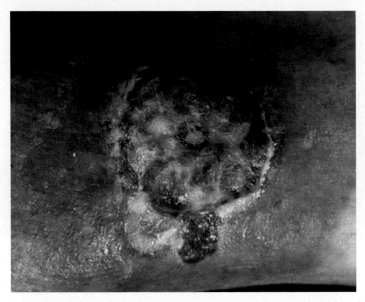

FIGURE 30-2. Well-circumscribed ulcerative yellow-red plaque with surrounding erythema arising in a chronic venous ulcer with background lipodermatosclerosis and stasis dermatitis on a lower extremity. (Reproduced with permission from Wolff K, Johnson RA, Saavedra AP, et al. *Fitzpatrick's Color Atlas and Synopsis of Clinical Dermatology*, 8th ed. New York, NY: McGraw Hill; 2017, Figure 17-12.)

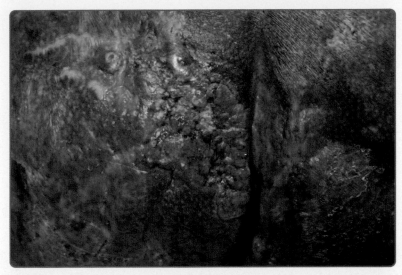

FIGURE 30-3. Ulcerated vegetative pink plaque representing a squamous cell carcinoma on the left buttock arising in a darker-skinned person with chronic inflammation secondary to hidradenitis suppurativa. (Reproduced with permission from Kang S, Amagai M, Bruckner AL, et al. *Fitzpatrick's Dermatology*, 9th ed. New York, NY: McGraw Hill; 2019, Figure 84-8.)

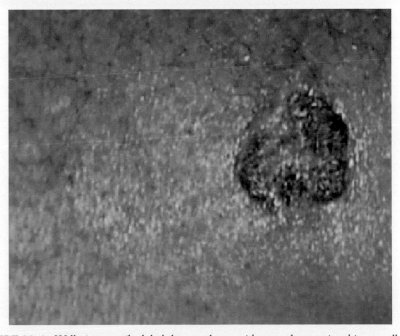

FIGURE 30-4. Well-circumscribed dark-brown plaque with normal-appearing skin centrally, representing Bowen disease on the forearm of a Black man. (Reproduced with permission from Taylor SC, Kelly AP, Lim HW, et al. *Taylor and Kelly's Dermatology for Skin of Color*, 2nd ed. New York, NY: McGraw Hill; 2016, Figure 45-5.)

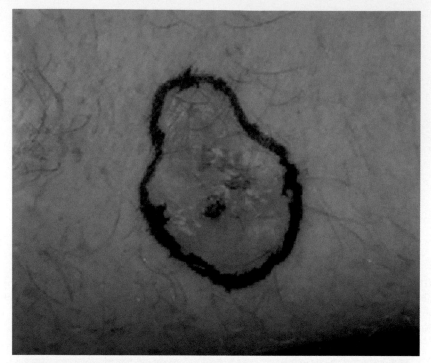

FIGURE 30-5. Well-demarcated pink scaly plaque with an overlying central scab on the forearm of a Hispanic woman. (Reproduced with permission from Taylor SC, Kelly AP, Lim HW, et al. *Taylor and Kelly's Dermatology for Skin of Color*, 2nd ed. New York, NY: McGraw Hill; 2016, Figure 45-7.)

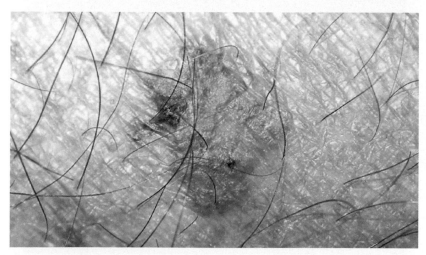

FIGURE 30-6. Well-circumscribed pink and brown plaque on the upper extremity. (From Usatine RP, Smith MA, Mayeaux EJ Jr, et al. *The Color Atlas and Synopsis of Family Medicine*, 3rd ed. New York, NY: McGraw Hill; 2019, Figure 173-7. Reproduced with permission from Richard P. Usatine, MD.)

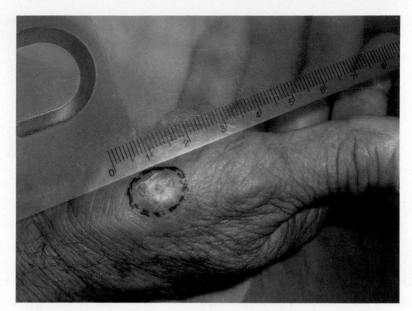

FIGURE 30-7. Pink-grey scaly plaque mimicking features of a basal cell carcinoma on the thenar eminence of the hand. (From Usatine RP, Smith MA, Mayeaux EJ Jr, et al. *The Color Atlas and Synopsis of Family Medicine*, 3rd ed. New York, NY: McGraw Hill; 2019, Figure 178-14. Reproduced with permission from Richard P. Usatine, MD.)

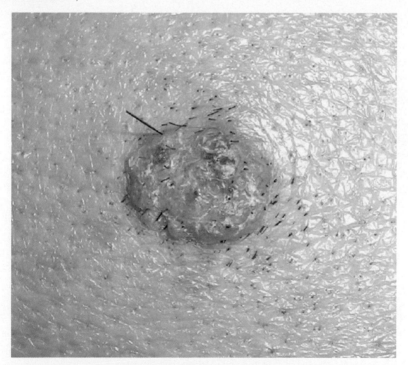

FIGURE 30-8. Well-circumscribed pink scaly plaque mimicking a verruca on the scalp. (From Usatine RP, Smith MA, Mayeaux EJ Jr, et al. *The Color Atlas and Synopsis of Family Medicine*, 3rd ed. New York, NY: McGraw Hill; 2019, Figure 178-11. Reproduced with permission from Richard P. Usatine, MD.)

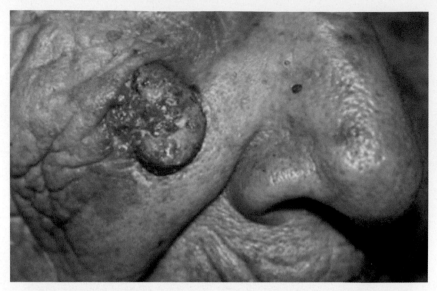

FIGURE 30-9. Light to dark-pink exophytic mass on the right cheek. (Reproduced with permission from Taylor SC, Kelly AP, Lim HW, et al. *Taylor and Kelly's Dermatology for Skin of Color*, 2nd ed. New York, NY: McGraw Hill; 2016, Figure 93A-16B.)

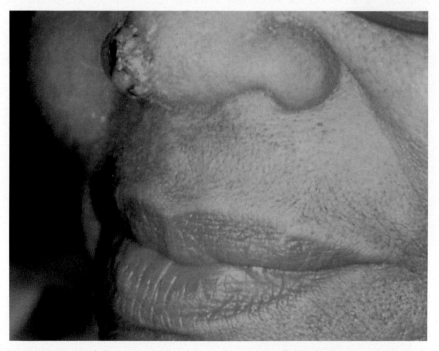

FIGURE 30-10. Pink-brown crusted papule on the nasal tip of a Black woman, mimicking a basal cell carcinoma. (Reproduced with permission from Taylor SC, Kelly AP, Lim HW, et al. *Taylor and Kelly's Dermatology for Skin of Color*, 2nd ed. New York, NY: McGraw Hill; 2016, Figure 45-1.)

KEY POINTS

- Melanoma in skin of color more commonly presents as acral lentiginous melanoma, which can be on palmar and plantar surfaces as well as nails.

- Other types of melanomas include superficial, nodular, ulcerative, and amelanotic.

- In skin of color, melanomas can mimic pigmented basal cell and pigmented seborrheic keratoses.

- Increased rates of delayed and missed diagnoses of melanomas in patients with skin of color contributes to advanced disease at time of presentation and increased morbidity and mortality.

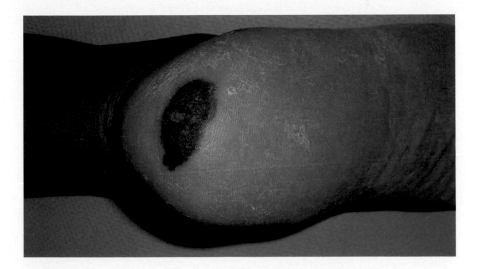

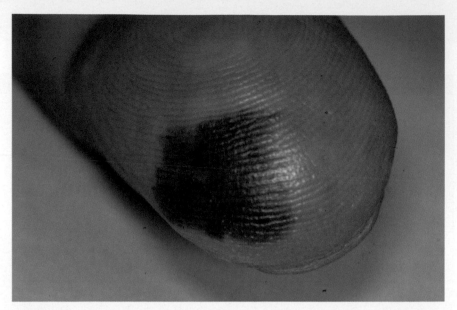

FIGURE 31-1. Dark-brown patch with irregular borders on the palmar surface of a Hispanic person. (Reproduced with permission from Taylor SC, Kelly AP, Lim HW, et al. *Taylor and Kelly's Dermatology for Skin of Color*, 2nd ed. New York, NY: McGraw Hill; 2016, Figure 19-4.)

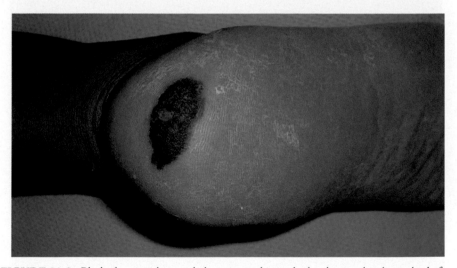

FIGURE 31-2. Black plaque with central ulceration and irregular borders on the plantar heel of a Black woman. (From Usatine RP, Smith MA, Mayeaux EJ Jr, et al. *The Color Atlas and Synopsis of Family Medicine*, 3rd ed. New York, NY: McGraw Hill; 2019, Figure 179-15. Reproduced with permission from Richard P. Usatine, MD.)

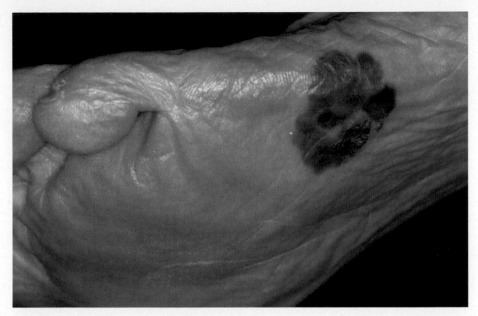

FIGURE 31-3. Dark-brown patch with variable colors, irregular borders, and an area of overlying superficial crusting. (Reproduced with permission from Soutor C, Hordinsky MK. *Clinical Dermatology.* New York, NY: McGraw Hill; 2013, Figure 18-13.)

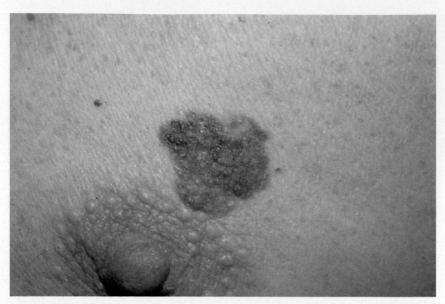

FIGURE 31-4. Pink, brown, and black plaque with irregular borders superior to the areola. (From Usatine RP, Smith MA, Mayeaux EJ Jr, et al. *The Color Atlas and Synopsis of Family Medicine*, 3rd ed. New York, NY: McGraw Hill; 2019, Figure 96-6. Reproduced with permission from Richard P. Usatine, MD.)

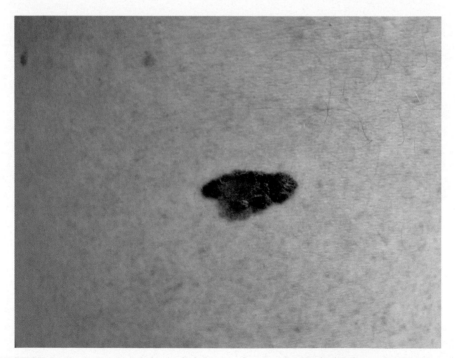

FIGURE 31-5. Asymmetric light- to dark-brown plaque with irregular borders and a raised papular component. (Reproduced with permission from Burgin S. *Guidebook to Dermatologic Diagnosis*. New York, NY: McGraw Hill; 2021, Figure 9-36.)

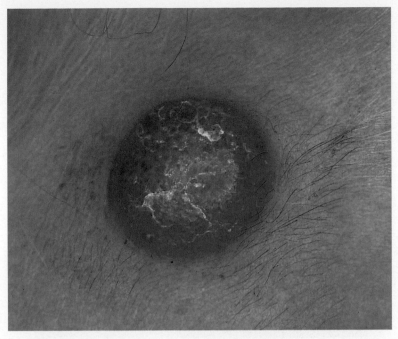

FIGURE 31-6. Pink, dome-shaped, scaly papule on the temple. (Reproduced with permission from Soutor C, Hordinsky MK. *Clinical Dermatology*. New York, NY: McGraw Hill; 2013, Figure 18-14.)

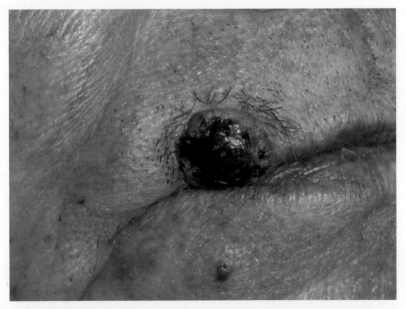

FIGURE 31-7. Multicolor nodule on the right lateral commissure. (From Usatine RP, Smith MA, Mayeaux EJ Jr, et al. *The Color Atlas and Synopsis of Family Medicine*, 3rd ed. New York, NY: McGraw Hill; 2019, Figure 179-7. Reproduced with permission from Jonathan B. Karnes, MD.)

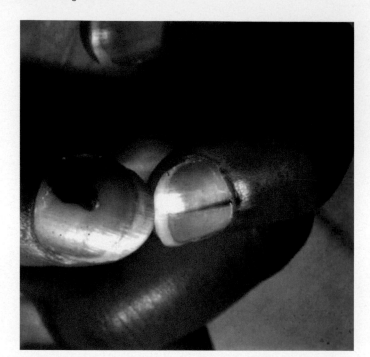

FIGURE 31-8. Linear light- to dark-brown streak on the third digit, which is wider at the base of the nail plate and extending onto the proximal nail fold. (Reproduced with permission from Taylor SC, Kelly AP, Lim HW, et al. *Taylor and Kelly's Dermatology for Skin of Color,* 2nd ed. New York, NY: McGraw Hill; 2016, Figure 44-5.)

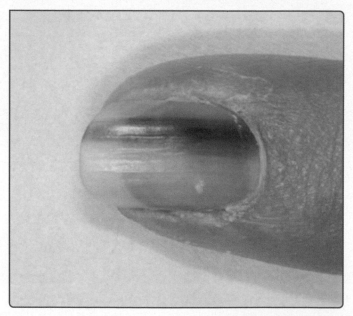

FIGURE 31-9. Tan to dark-brown linear streak with central darkening extending the full length of the nail plate. (Reproduced with permission from Kang S, Amagai M, Bruckner AL, et al. *Fitzpatrick's Dermatology,* 9th ed. New York, NY: McGraw Hill; 2019, Figure 116-2G.)

KEY POINTS

- Mycosis fungoides (MF) can present with multiple variants including hypopigmented, folliculotropic, pagetoid reticulosis, granulomatous slack skin, and Sézary syndrome.

- Hypopigmented MF is a variant seen more commonly in skin of color. It can be mistaken for atopic dermatitis and pityriasis alba when on the face. This can also contribute to delays in diagnosis and increased disease morbidity.

- MF can also present as hyperpigmented patches and can often resolve with dyspigmentation.

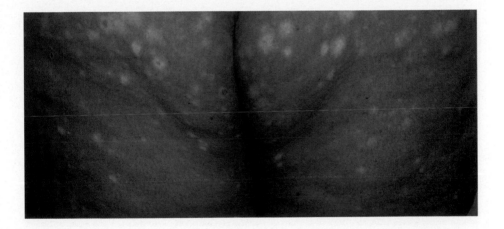

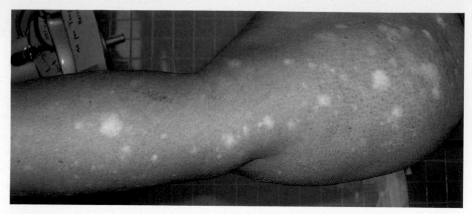

FIGURE 32-1. Numerous scattered, nummular, hypopigmented macules and patches, some of which appear almost depigmented, on the right ventral upper extremity. The depigmented-appearing patches may mimic the appearance of vitiligo. (From Usatine RP, Smith MA, Mayeaux EJ Jr, et al. *The Color Atlas and Synopsis of Family Medicine*, 3rd ed. New York, NY: McGraw Hill; 2019, Figure 180-2. Reproduced with permission from Richard P. Usatine, MD.)

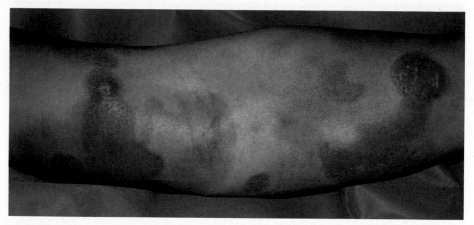

FIGURE 32-2. Red patches and plaques with areas of overlying scale and peripheral background light-brown patches. (Reproduced with permission from Kane KS, Nambudiri VE, Stratigos AJ. *Color Atlas & Synopsis of Pediatric Dermatology*, 3rd ed. New York, NY: McGraw Hill; 2017, Figure 19-9.)

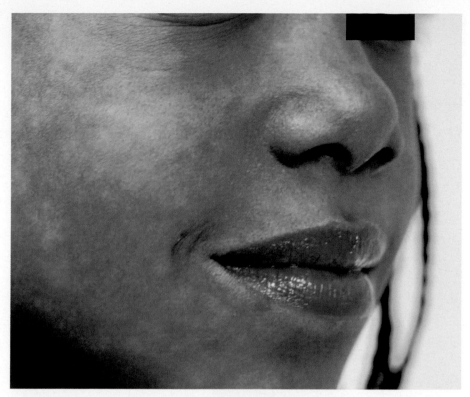

FIGURE 32-3. Ill-defined hypopigmented macules coalescing into patches without overlying scale on the face of a young female. This presentation is similar to what can also be seen in pityriasis alba. (Reproduced with permission from Prose NS, Kristal L. *Weinberg's Color Atlas of Pediatric Dermatology*, 5th ed. New York, NY: McGraw Hill; 2017, Figure 12-45.)

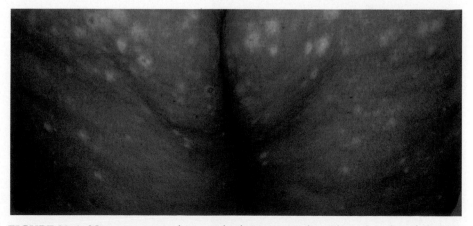

FIGURE 32-4. Numerous scattered, nummular, hypopigmented macules and patches of varying size, with mild background erythema on the bilateral anterior thighs. (From Usatine RP, Smith MA, Mayeaux EJ Jr, et al. *The Color Atlas and Synopsis of Family Medicine*, 3rd ed. New York, NY: McGraw Hill; 2019, Figure 180-1. Reproduced with permission from Richard P. Usatine, MD.)

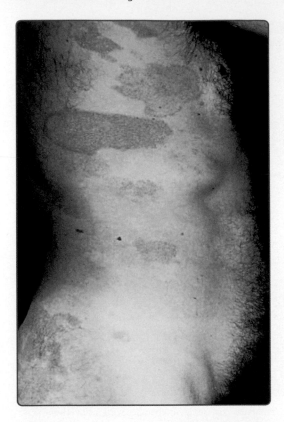

FIGURE 32-5. Large red-orange patches and plaques on the lateral trunk and buttock, representing cutaneous T-cell lymphoma stage IB. (Reproduced with permission from Kang S, Amagai M, Bruckner AL, et al. *Fitzpatrick's Dermatology*, 9th ed. New York, NY: McGraw Hill; 2019, Figure 199-5A.)

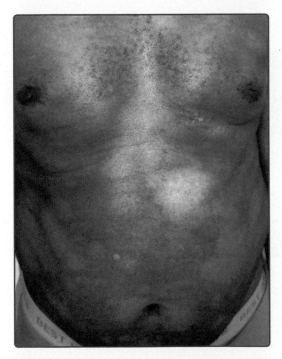

FIGURE 32-6. Ill-defined large hypopigmented patches on the anterior trunk. Note the lack of visible scale. (Reproduced with permission from Kang S, Amagai M, Bruckner AL, et al. *Fitzpatrick's Dermatology*, 9th ed. New York, NY: McGraw Hill; 2019, Figure 76-16.)

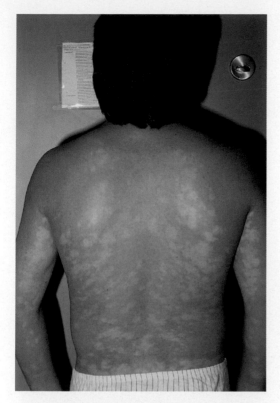

FIGURE 32-7. Large hypopigmented patches on the posterior trunk and upper extremities in a seborrheic distribution mimicking the presentation of pityriasis rosea in a Latinx person. (Reproduced with permission from Taylor SC, Kelly AP, Lim HW, et al. *Taylor and Kelly's Dermatology for Skin of Color*, 2nd ed. New York, NY: McGraw Hill; 2016, Figure 47-1.)

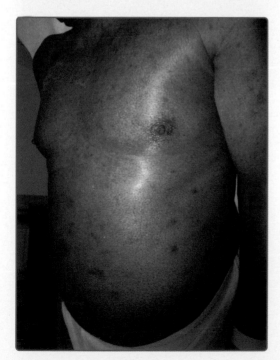

FIGURE 32-8. Scattered dark-brown patches and plaques on the anterior trunk and upper extremities representing cutaneous T-cell leukemia/lymphoma. (From Kang S, Amagai M, Bruckner AL, et al. *Fitzpatrick's Dermatology*, 9th ed. New York, NY: McGraw Hill; 2019, Figure 168-15. Reproduced with permission from Dr. Thomas Kupper and Marianne Tawa, NP.)

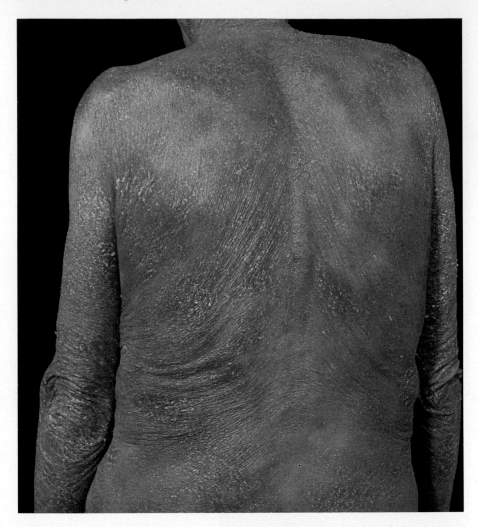

FIGURE 32-9. Large red, scaly, and desquamating lichenified patches with areas of sparing diffusely on the posterior trunk and upper extremities, representing Sézary syndrome. (Reproduced with permission from Wolff K, Johnson RA, Saavedra AP, et al. *Fitzpatrick's Color Atlas and Synopsis of Clinical Dermatology*, 8th ed. New York, NY: McGraw Hill; 2017, Figure 8-3.)

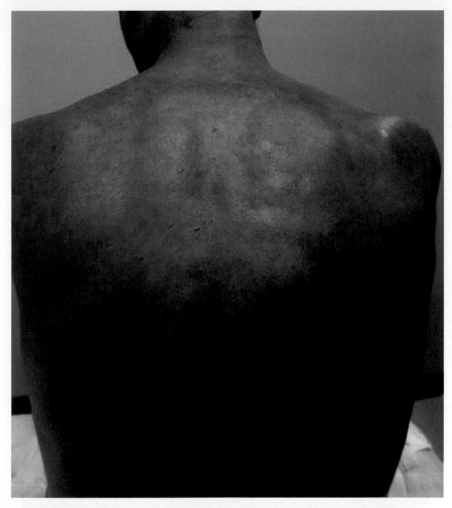

FIGURE 32-10. Posterior trunk of a Black man with Sézary syndrome, showing diffuse erythroderma most notable at the periphery of areas of sparing. (Reproduced with permission from Jackson-Richards D, Pandya AG. *Dermatology Atlas for Skin of Color.* Berlin Heidelberg: Springer-Verlag; 2014.)

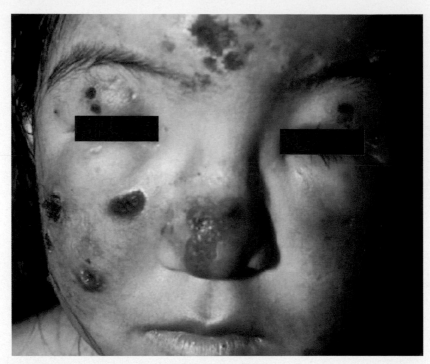

FIGURE 32-11. Red ulcerative vesicles and plaques with areas of overlying crusting in the setting of background facial edema representing the hydroa vacciniforme-like cutaneous T-cell lymphoma variant. (Reproduced with permission from Prose NS, Kristal L. *Weinberg's Color Atlas of Pediatric Dermatology*, 5th ed. New York, NY: McGraw Hill; 2017, Figure 24-21.)

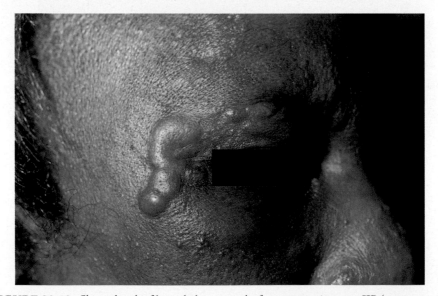

FIGURE 32-12. Skin-colored infiltrated plaques on the face representing stage IIB (tumor stage) cutaneous T-cell lymphoma. (Reproduced with permission from Taylor SC, Kelly AP, Lim HW, et al. *Taylor and Kelly's Dermatology for Skin of Color*, 2nd ed. New York, NY: McGraw Hill; 2016, Figure 47-4.)

Pigmentary Disorders

KEY POINTS

- Longitudinal melanonychia (LM) is a benign presentation of vertical pigmented streaks on the nail plate that typically range in color from tan to dark brown.

- LM is more common in skin of color, and those with melanonychia should be evaluated to rule out acral melanoma.

- Its presence in multiple digits can help confirm the diagnosis of melanonychia and decreases the likelihood of melanoma.

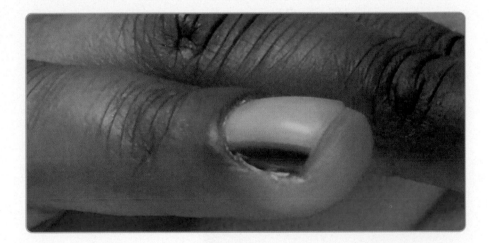

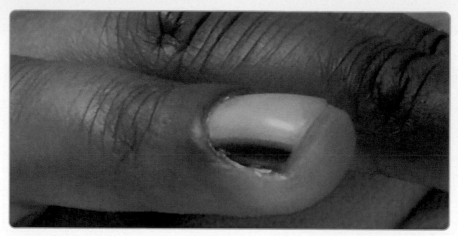

FIGURE 33-1. Dark-brown linear streak with darker central pigmentation, secondary to a matrix lentigo, extending along the full length of the lateral nail plate of a dark-skinned individual. (Reproduced with permission from Kang S, Amagai M, Bruckner AL, et al. *Fitzpatrick's Dermatology*, 9th ed. New York, NY: McGraw Hill; 2019, Figure 91-82.)

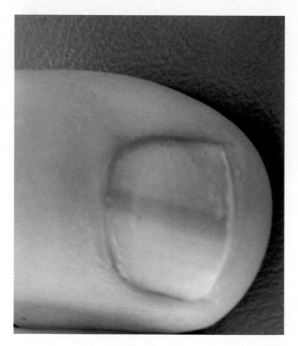

FIGURE 33-2. Light-brown–gray linear streak located centrally on the nail plate of the great toe of a person with light skin. (Reproduced with permission from Taylor SC, Kelly AP, Lim HW, et al. *Taylor and Kelly's Dermatology for Skin of Color*, 2nd ed. New York, NY: McGraw Hill; 2016, Figure 40-2.)

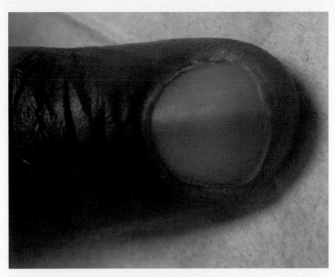

FIGURE 33-3. Faint light-brown central linear streak on the nail plate of a dark-skinned person, demonstrating the variability in the intensity of color that can be seen in people with dark skin. (Reproduced with permission from Taylor SC, Kelly AP, Lim HW, et al. *Taylor and Kelly's Dermatology for Skin of Color*, 2nd ed. New York, NY: McGraw Hill; 2016, Figure 21-3.)

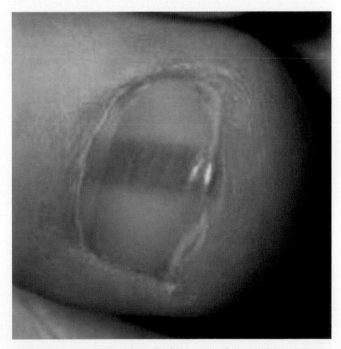

FIGURE 33-4. Tan linear streak extending the full length of the nail plate on a person with lighter skin. (Reproduced with permission from Prose NS, Kristal L. *Weinberg's Color Atlas of Pediatric Dermatology*, 5th ed. New York, NY: McGraw Hill; 2017, Figure 26-11.)

KEY POINTS

- Melasma occurs more commonly in women and though it can occur in all skin colors it is more common in those darker skin tones.

- Facial melasma has three distributions that include centrofacial, malar, and mandibular. Extrafacial melasma can also occur less commonly on non-facial sites.

- Melasma can vary in distribution and severity, with color ranging from tan to dark brown.

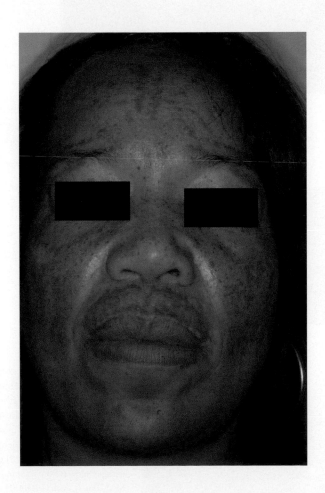

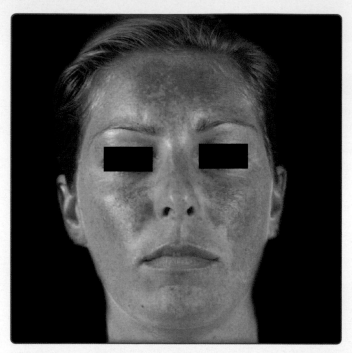

FIGURE 34-1. Tan to dark-brown patches with central areas of sparing located on the forehead, cheeks, and chin of a young White woman. (Reproduced with permission from Kang S, Amagai M, Bruckner AL, et al. *Fitzpatrick's Dermatology*, 9th ed. New York, NY: McGraw Hill; 2019, Figure 137-13.)

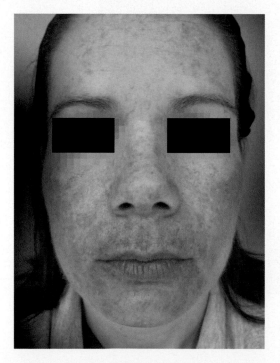

FIGURE 34-2. Large, diffuse, tan-brown symmetric patches with areas of subtle background erythema more densely located on the cheeks, upper cutaneous lip, and chin, along with lateral forehead involvement, in a young woman with light skin. (Reproduced with permission from Tannous Z, Avram MM, Tsao S, et al. *Color Atlas of Cosmetic Dermatology*, 2nd ed. New York, NY: McGraw Hill; 2011, Figure 5-1.)

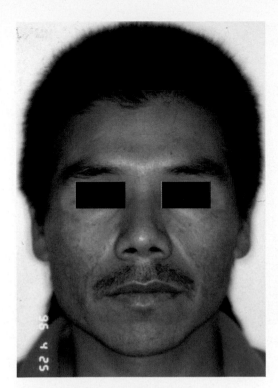

FIGURE 34-3. Medium-brown macules and patches symmetrically located on the cheeks, along with the forehead and chin, of a Latin American man. (Reproduced with permission from Taylor SC, Kelly AP, Lim HW, et al. *Taylor and Kelly's Dermatology for Skin of Color*, 2nd ed. New York, NY: McGraw Hill; 2016, Figure 51-5.)

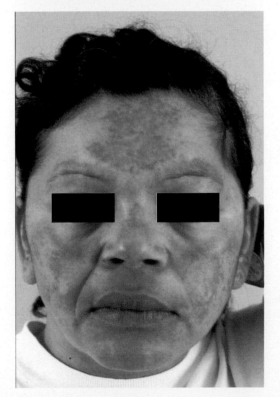

FIGURE 34-4. Prominent, medium-brown reticulated patches on the central forehead, cheeks, and perioral skin of a woman of color. (Reproduced with permission from Taylor SC, Kelly AP, Lim HW, et al. *Taylor and Kelly's Dermatology for Skin of Color*, 2nd ed. New York, NY: McGraw Hill; 2016, Figure 51-4.)

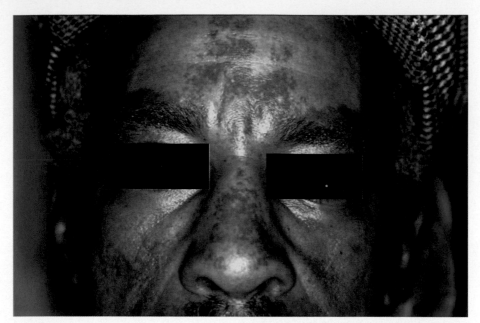

FIGURE 34-5. Dark-brown patches with irregular borders in a centrofacial pattern in a Black man. (Reproduced with permission from Taylor SC, Kelly AP, Lim HW, et al. *Taylor and Kelly's Dermatology for Skin of Color*, 2nd ed. New York, NY: McGraw Hill; 2016, Figure 51-3.)

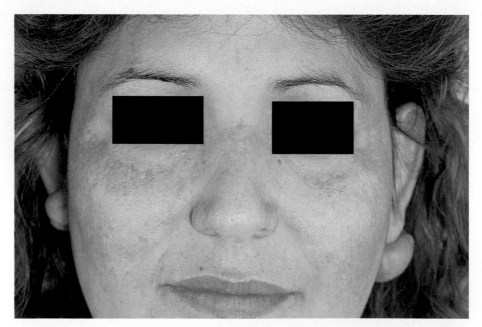

FIGURE 34-6. Tan, ill-defined, reticulated symmetric patches along the lateral cheeks of a Hispanic woman, with sparing of the mid-cheek region. (Reproduced with permission from Taylor SC, Kelly AP, Lim HW, et al. *Taylor and Kelly's Dermatology for Skin of Color*, 2nd ed. New York, NY: McGraw Hill; 2016, Figure 51-2.)

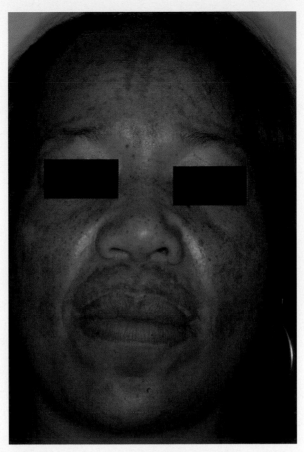

FIGURE 34-7. Medium- to dark-brown patches and streaks with irregular borders on the forehead (including eyebrows), cheeks, upper cutaneous lip, and chin of a woman of color. (Reproduced with permission from Taylor SC, Kelly AP, Lim HW, et al. *Taylor and Kelly's Dermatology for Skin of Color*, 2nd ed. New York, NY: McGraw Hill; 2016, Figure 78-1A.)

KEY POINTS

- Postinflammatory pigment alteration (PIPA) includes both postinflammatory hyperpigmentation and postinflammatory hypopigmentation.

- While PIPA can occur in all skin colors, it is more common in skin of color.

- Individuals affected with PIPA are thought to have a predisposed tendency for their melanocytes to respond to inflammation or trauma with hyperpigmentation or hypopigmentation.

- PIPA can often last significantly longer than the underlying cause. It has been associated with profound effects on quality of life.

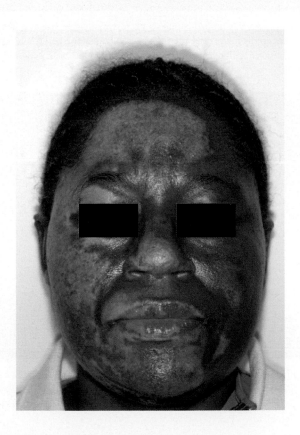

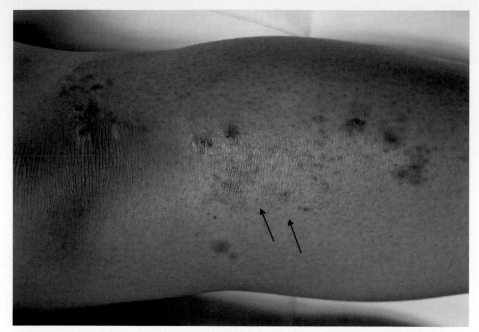

FIGURE 35-1. Violaceous flat-topped papules with surrounding erythema and brown macules coalescing into patches on the lower extremity of a person with active and resolving lichen planus. (Reproduced with permission from Burgin S. *Guidebook to Dermatologic Diagnosis*. New York, NY: McGraw Hill; 2021, Figure 3-28.)

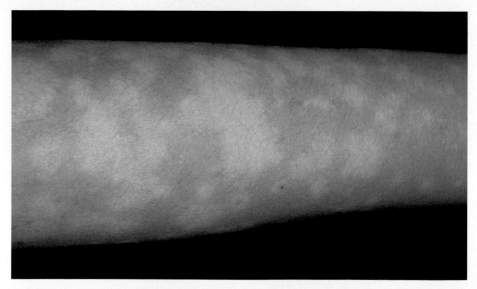

FIGURE 35-2. Hypopigmented patches with background areas of erythema in a light-skinned person treated for psoriasis. (From Usatine RP, Smith MA, Mayeaux EJ Jr, et al. *The Color Atlas and Synopsis of Family Medicine*, 3rd ed. New York, NY: McGraw Hill; 2019, Figure 110-21. Reproduced with permission from Richard P. Usatine, MD.)

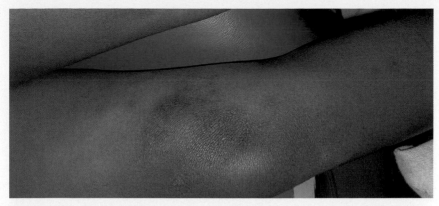

FIGURE 35-3. Violaceous to dark-brown patches along the knees and medial thigh of a young Black person, signifying postinflammatory hyperpigmentation secondary to atopic dermatitis. (From Usatine RP, Smith MA, Mayeaux EJ Jr, et al. *The Color Atlas and Synopsis of Family Medicine*, 3rd ed. New York, NY: McGraw Hill; 2019, Figure 207-1B. Reproduced with permission from Richard P. Usatine, MD.)

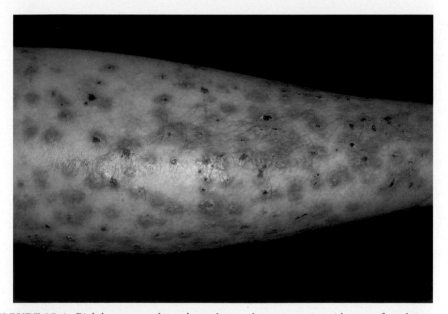

FIGURE 35-4. Pink-brown macules and papules on a lower extremity, with areas of overlying excoriations signifying postinflammatory erythema and hyperpigmentation in a person with light skin. (From Usatine RP, Smith MA, Mayeaux EJ Jr, et al. *The Color Atlas and Synopsis of Family Medicine*, 3rd ed. New York, NY: McGraw Hill; 2019, Figure 155-4. Reproduced with permission from Richard P. Usatine, MD.)

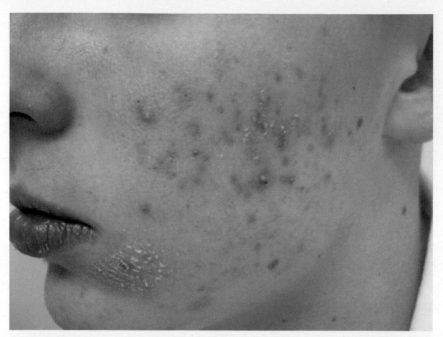

FIGURE 35-5. Pink macules and papules on the left cheek of a young light-skinned patient with acne. (Reproduced with permission from Alam M, Bhatia AC, Kundu RV, et al. *Cosmetic Dermatology for Skin of Color.* New York, NY: McGraw Hill; 2009, Figure 17-2.)

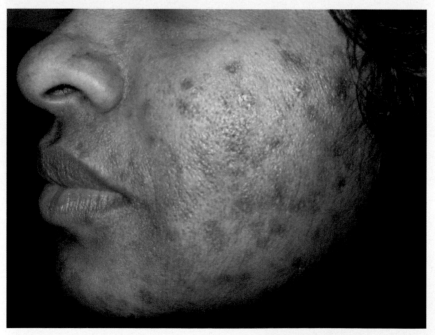

FIGURE 35-6. Light to brown macules on the cheeks, jawline, and perioral skin consistent with postinflammatory hyperpigmentation secondary to acne. Note the lack of active acne. (Reproduced with permission from Alam M, Bhatia AC, Kundu RV, et al. *Cosmetic Dermatology for Skin of Color.* New York, NY: McGraw Hill; 2009, Figure 18-4.)

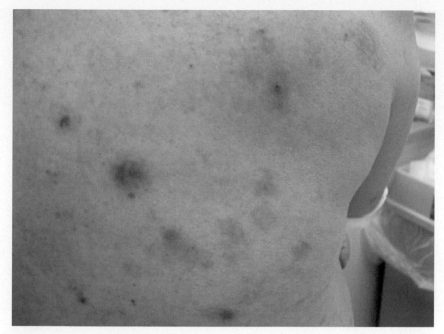

FIGURE 35-7. Pink and brown patches secondary to nummular eczema, scattered on the back of an Asian man. (Reproduced with permission from Alam M, Bhatia AC, Kundu RV, et al. *Cosmetic Dermatology for Skin of Color.* New York, NY: McGraw Hill; 2009, Figure 17-1.)

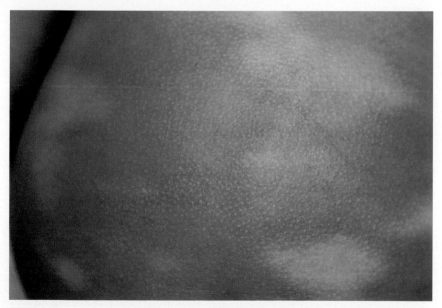

FIGURE 35-8. Ill-defined hypopigmented patches on the abdomen of a young child secondary to a resolved inflammatory disease. (Reproduced with permission from Prose NS, Kristal L. *Weinberg's Color Atlas of Pediatric Dermatology,* 5th ed. New York, NY: McGraw Hill; 2017, Figure 27-21.)

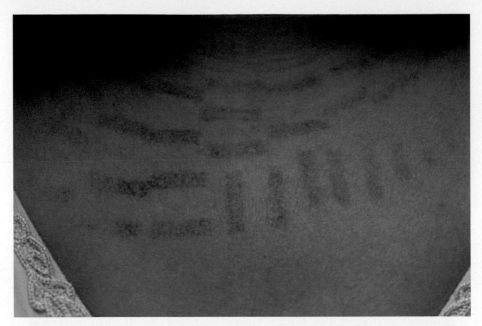

FIGURE 35-9. Brown rectangular patches on the anterior chest of a Black woman secondary to laser hair removal. (Reproduced with permission from Taylor SC, Kelly AP, Lim HW, et al. *Taylor and Kelly's Dermatology for Skin of Color*, 2nd ed. New York, NY: McGraw Hill; 2016, Figure 52-5.)

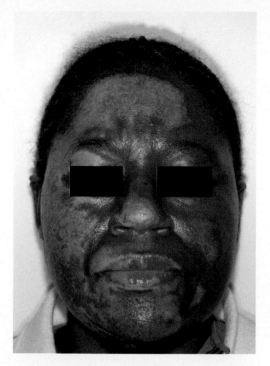

FIGURE 35-10. Large hypopigmented patches on the face secondary to a burn from a chemical peel. Note the brown areas within the hypopigmentation signifying areas of repigmentation. (Reproduced with permission from Taylor SC, Kelly AP, Lim HW, et al. *Taylor and Kelly's Dermatology for Skin of Color,* 2nd ed. New York, NY: McGraw Hill; 2016, Figure 78-3.)

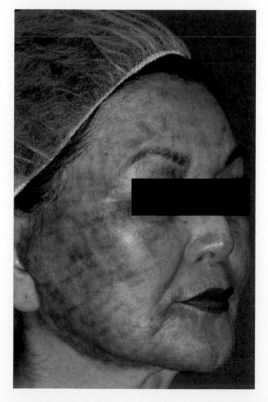

FIGURE 35-11. Linear brown streaks diffusely present on the face of an Asian woman with Fitzpatrick type IV skin secondary to fractional CO_2 laser treatment. (Reproduced with permission from Avram MR, Avram MM, Ratner D. *Procedural Dermatology.* New York, NY: McGraw Hill; 2015, Figure 35-9A.)

Photosensitive Disorders

CHAPTER 36 ▪ POLYMORPHOUS LIGHT ERUPTION

KEY POINTS

- Polymorphous light eruption (PMLE) can present with various morphologies in photoexposed areas including papular, papulosquamous, and urticarial.

- Color can vary across skin types. In skin of color, PMLE can present as skin colored to pink or violaceous. In lighter skin, it can be vary from faint pink to bright red.

- Presentation can mimic systemic lupus erythematous on the face.

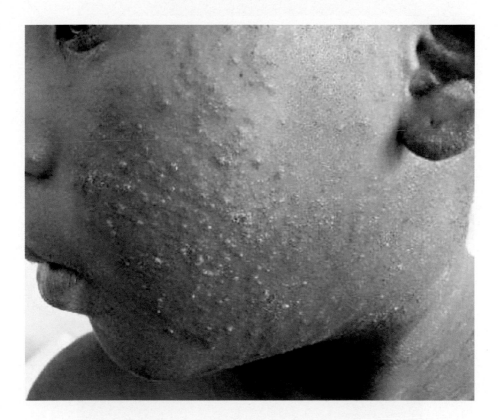

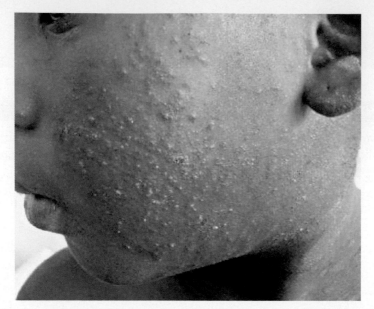

FIGURE 36-1. Pinpoint white papules with areas of scaling and crusting overlying a background of erythema on the left cheek in a young Black boy. Note the involvement of the left earlobe and neck as well as the background hyperpigmentation in these locations. (Reproduced with permission from Prose NS, Kristal L. *Weinberg's Color Atlas of Pediatric Dermatology*, 5th ed. New York, NY: McGraw Hill; 2017, Figure 11-4.)

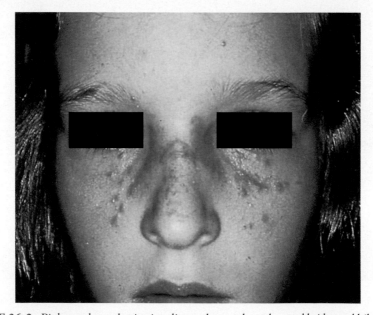

FIGURE 36-2. Pink papules coalescing into linear plaques along the nasal bridge and bilateral cheeks of a young woman, mimicking the butterfly rash of another photosensitive disorder, systemic lupus erythematosus. (Reproduced with permission from Prose NS, Kristal L. *Weinberg's Color Atlas of Pediatric Dermatology*, 5th ed. New York, NY: McGraw Hill; 2017, Figure 11-3.)

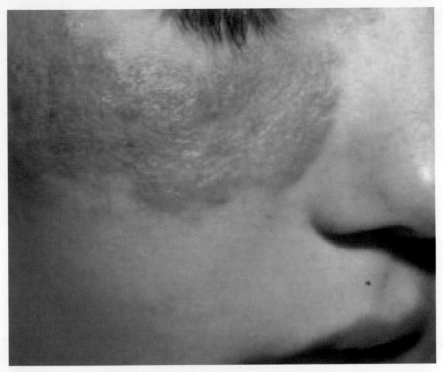

FIGURE 36-3. Well-demarcated pink edematous plaque on the right malar cheek of an indigenous child. (Reproduced with permission from Prose NS, Kristal L. *Weinberg's Color Atlas of Pediatric Dermatology*, 5th ed. New York, NY: McGraw Hill; 2017, Figure 11-2.)

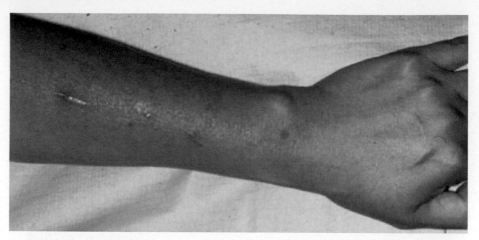

FIGURE 36-4. Pinpoint skin-colored papules on the dorsal forearms. (Reproduced with permission from Taylor SC, Kelly AP, Lim HW, et al. *Taylor and Kelly's Dermatology for Skin of Color*, 2nd ed. New York, NY: McGraw Hill; 2016, Figure 29-2A.)

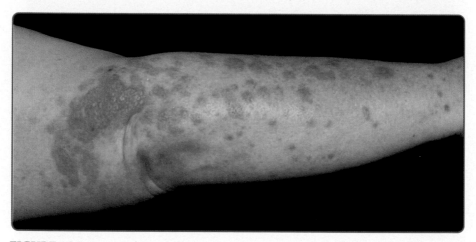

FIGURE 36-5. Large pink urticarial plaques on the extensor forearm of a young man. (Reproduced with permission from Kang S, Amagai M, Bruckner AL, et al. *Fitzpatrick's Dermatology*, 9th ed. New York, NY: McGraw Hill; 2019, Figure 92-5D.)

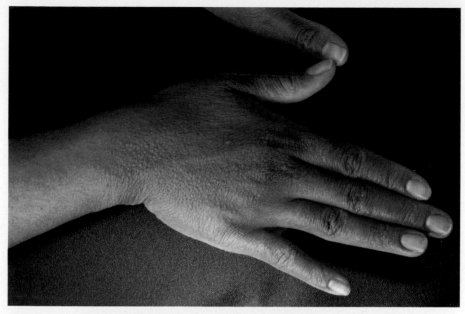

FIGURE 36-6. Fine, skin-colored, confluent papules on the dorsal hand. Note the lack of visible erythema. (Reproduced with permission from Taylor SC, Kelly AP, Lim HW, et al. *Taylor and Kelly's Dermatology for Skin of Color*, 2nd ed. New York, NY: McGraw Hill; 2016, Figure 29-1.)

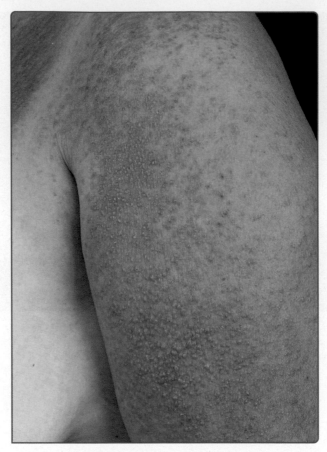

FIGURE 36-7. Diffuse, confluent, pink, pinpoint papules on the left upper extremity. Note the sparing of the non–sun-exposed areas. (Reproduced with permission from Kang S, Amagai M, Bruckner AL, et al. *Fitzpatrick's Dermatology*, 9th ed. New York, NY: McGraw Hill; 2019, Figure 92-3B.)

KEY POINTS

- Chronic actinic dermatitis presents with a well-demarcated eczematous dermatitis consisting of scaly, pruritic patches and plaques confined to the head and neck.

- In lighter skin, this can vary from pink to red erythema, while in darker skin, it can be pink-brown to violaceous to brown-black.

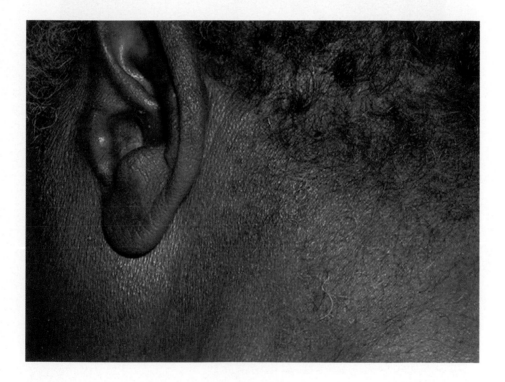

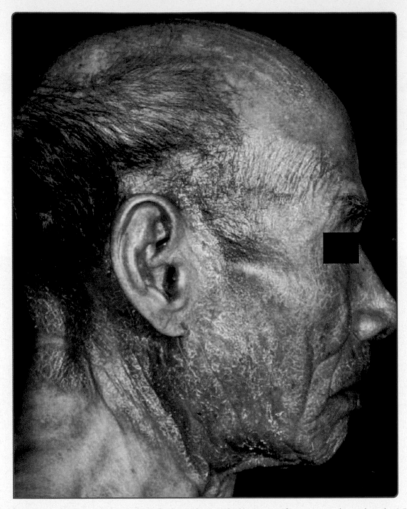

FIGURE 37-1. Pink-tan scaly lichenified patches and plaques on face, ear, neck, and scalp. Note the sparing of the neck fold. (Reproduced with permission from Kang S, Amagai M, Bruckner AL, et al. *Fitzpatrick's Dermatology*, 9th ed. New York, NY: McGraw Hill; 2019, Figure 95-2A.)

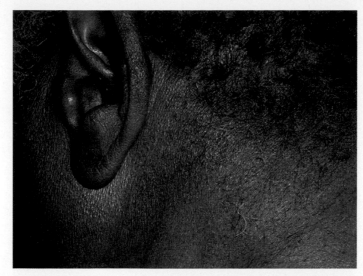

FIGURE 37-2. Violaceous-brown patches on the lateral cheek, ear, and posterior neck with background postinflammatory hyperpigmentation from chronic actinic dermatitis in a Black male. (Reproduced with permission from Silpa-Archa N, Kohli I, Chaowattanapanit S, et al. Postinflammatory hyperpigmentation: A comprehensive overview: Epidemiology, pathogenesis, clinical presentation, and noninvasive assessment technique. *J Am Acad Dermatol.* 2017;77(4):591-605.)

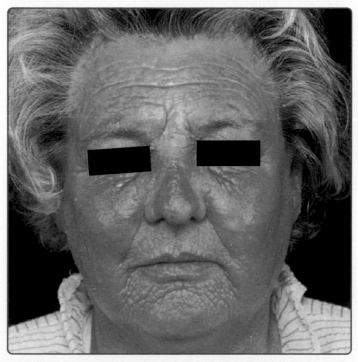

FIGURE 37-3. Diffuse erythema and edema on the face with visible infiltrated skin-colored plaques on the chin. (Reproduced with permission from Kang S, Amagai M, Bruckner AL, et al. *Fitzpatrick's Dermatology*, 9th ed. New York, NY: McGraw Hill; 2019, Figure 95-1.)

Drug Reactions

KEY POINTS

- Morbilliform eruptions tend to present with diffuse papules coalescing into plaques.
- In darker skin, these papules are often violaceous to dark brown with minimal to no visible background erythema.
- In contrast, lighter skin tends to show bright pink to red papules with a marked background of erythema.
- In both cases, there can be little to no sparing of normal skin.

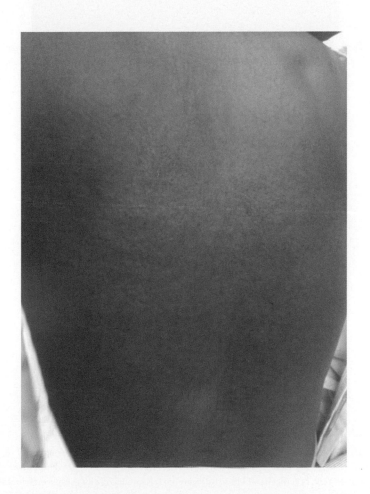

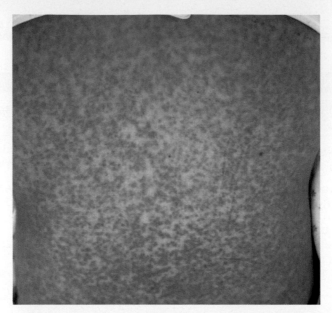

FIGURE 38-1. Diffuse and densely scattered bright-pink macules and confluent papules on the back. (Reproduced with permission from Burgin S. *Guidebook to Dermatologic Diagnosis*. New York, NY: McGraw Hill; 2021, Figure 10-13.)

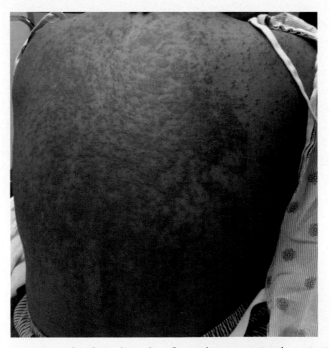

FIGURE 38-2. Magenta-colored papules and confluent plaques covering the majority of the back in a person of color. (From Taylor SC, Kelly AP, Lim HW, et al. *Taylor and Kelly's Dermatology for Skin of Color*, 2nd ed. New York, NY: McGraw Hill; 2016, Figure 35-1. Reproduced with permission from Lisa Pappas-Taffer, MD.)

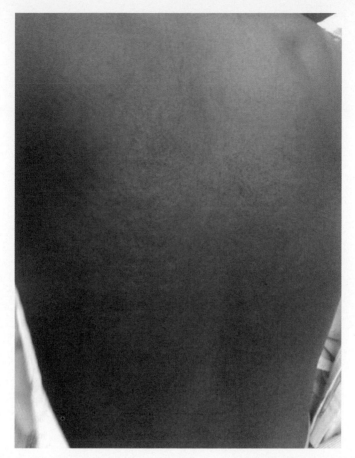

FIGURE 38-3. Densely scattered violaceous and brown macules and papules over a background of subtle erythema in a person with dark skin. (From Taylor SC, Kelly AP, Lim HW, et al. *Taylor and Kelly's Dermatology for Skin of Color*, 2nd ed. New York, NY: McGraw Hill; 2016, Figure 35-3. Reproduced with permission from Lisa Pappas-Taffer, MD.)

KEY POINTS

- Fixed drug eruption presents with well-demarcated nummular patches and plaques that vary in color across skin types.

- In darker skin, the patches and plaques tend to be dark brown to gray centrally with a peripheral rim that is lighter in color and ranges from magenta to violaceous.

- In lighter skin, the same morphology can range from bright pink to red centrally with a faint pink periphery.

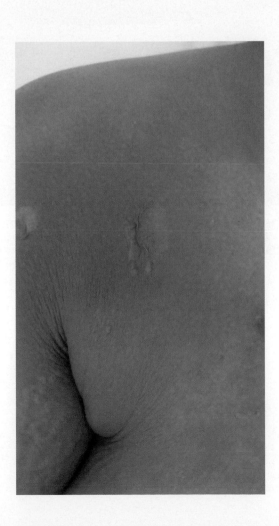

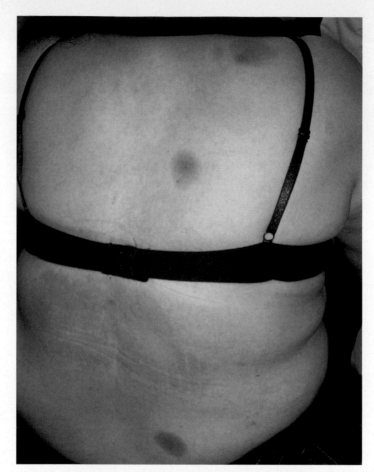

FIGURE 39-1. Discrete, nummular brown-gray patches on the back of a Hispanic woman. (From Usatine RP, Smith MA, Mayeaux EJ Jr, et al. *The Color Atlas and Synopsis of Family Medicine*, 3rd ed. New York, NY: McGraw Hill; 2019, Figure 212-20. Reproduced with permission from Richard P. Usatine, MD.)

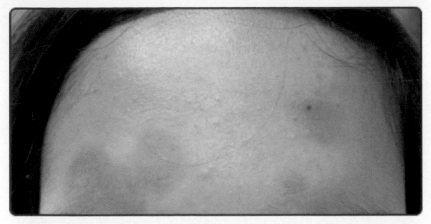

FIGURE 39-2. Light-brown–gray nummular patches on the forehead of Sri Lankan woman. (Reproduced with permission from Kang S, Amagai M, Bruckner AL, et al. *Fitzpatrick's Dermatology*, 9th ed. New York, NY: McGraw Hill; 2019, Figure 77-12.)

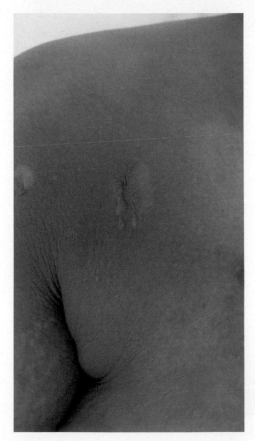

FIGURE 39-3. Dusky violaceous patches with a surrounding rim of erythema on the anterior trunk. (Reproduced with permission from Burgin S. *Guidebook to Dermatologic Diagnosis.* New York, NY: McGraw Hill; 2021, Figure 4-15.)

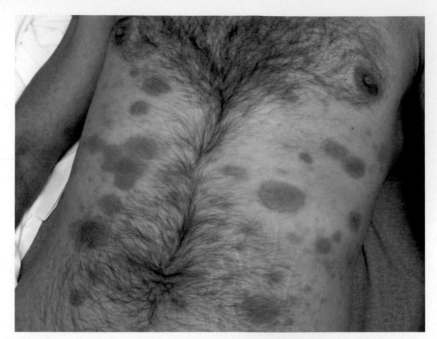

FIGURE 39-4. Bright-pink patches with dusky darker centers scattered across the anterior trunk of a person with a disseminated fixed drug reaction. (From Usatine RP, Smith MA, Mayeaux EJ Jr, et al. *The Color Atlas and Synopsis of Family Medicine*, 3rd ed. New York, NY: McGraw Hill; 2019, Figure 212-9. Reproduced with permission from Bucher J, Rahnama-Moghadam S, Osswald S. Generalized rash follows ankle ulceration. *J Fam Pract.* 2016;65(7):489-491.)

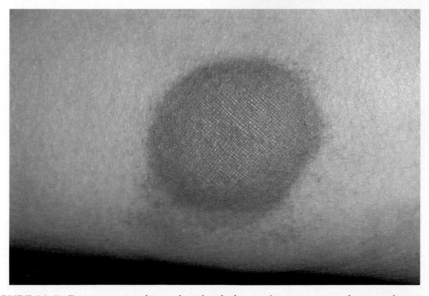

FIGURE 39-5. Discrete nummular patch with a dusky purple-gray center and surrounding rim of bright-pink to purple erythema. (From Usatine RP, Smith MA, Mayeaux EJ Jr, et al. *The Color Atlas and Synopsis of Family Medicine*, 3rd ed. New York, NY: McGraw Hill; 2019, Figure 212-8. Reproduced with permission from Richard P. Usatine, MD.)

KEY POINTS

- Stevens-Johnson Syndrome (SJS) and toxic epidermal necrolysis (TEN) can appear differently across skin types in earlier stages of the diseases prior to the skin becoming denuded.

- In lighter skin, affected areas can be salmon colored to pink, while in darker skin, they can be violaceous to gray or gray-brown.

- In both skin types, hemorrhagic bullae and crusting can be seen along with erosions.

- In darker skin, areas will typically heal with postinflammatory dyspigmentation.

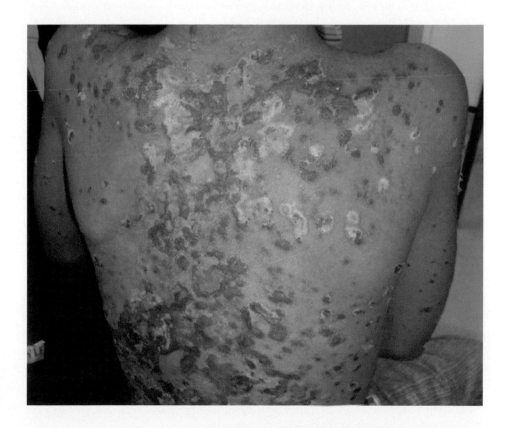

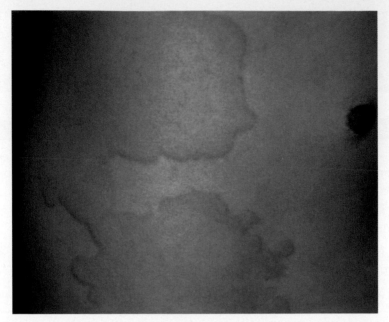

FIGURE 40-1. Diffuse salmon-red papules and confluent scaly patches and plaques with minimal areas of sparing on the neck, anterior trunk, and upper extremities. (Reproduced with permission from Prose NS, Kristal L. *Weinberg's Color Atlas of Pediatric Dermatology*, 5th ed. New York, NY: McGraw Hill; 2017, Figure 16-3.)

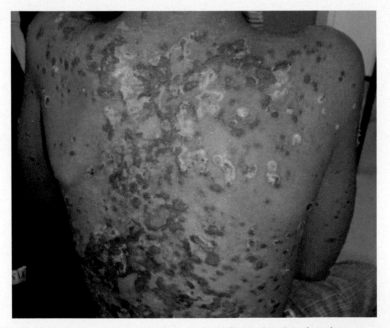

FIGURE 40-2. Violaceous scaly papules and plaques diffusely distributed on the posterior trunk with numerous areas of bright-pink denuded skin, several of which are also hemorrhagic on the lower back. (Reproduced with permission from Prose NS, Kristal L. *Weinberg's Color Atlas of Pediatric Dermatology*, 5th ed. New York, NY: McGraw Hill; 2017, Figure 18-5.)

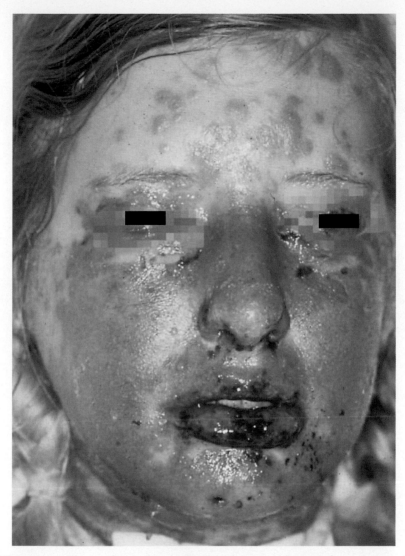

FIGURE 40-3. Diffuse confluent salmon-colored patches on an edematous face with areas of hemorrhagic crusting on the eyelids, lips, nose, and periocular and perioral skin. Note the areas of sparing on the forehead and neck, which primarily have salmon-colored papules and plaques. (Reproduced with permission from Soutor C, Hordinsky MK. *Clinical Dermatology*. New York, NY: McGraw Hill; 2013, Figure 23-6.)

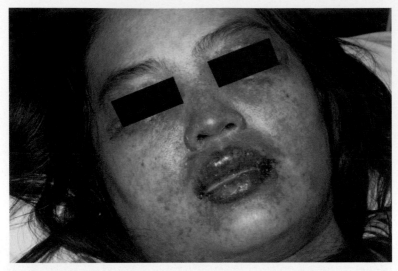

FIGURE 40-4. Diffuse pink macules and papules on the face of a young woman with overlying hemorrhagic crusting periocularly and periorally. Note the edema of the face and lips and the erosion inferior to the right nasal ala. (Reproduced with permission from Barnhill RL, Crowson AN, Magro CM, et al. *Barnhill's Dermatopathology*, 4th ed. New York, NY: McGraw Hill; 2020, Figure 8-21A.)

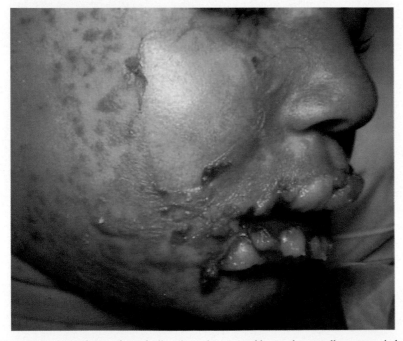

FIGURE 40-5. Intact hemorrhagic bullae along the mucosal lips and periorally, surrounded on the face by a large patch of denuded skin on the right cheek and peripheral brown patches. Note the lack of redness and erythema visible in this person who also has active SJS/TEN. (Reproduced with permission from Prose NS, Kristal L. *Weinberg's Color Atlas of Pediatric Dermatology*, 5th ed. New York, NY: McGraw Hill; 2017, Figure 16-17.)

KEY POINTS

- Erythema multiforme shares the same morphologic appearance across skin types, including a targetoid plaque with a central patch or bullae, but overall varies in color in different skin types.

- In darker skin, it can be pink-brown to violaceous to dark brown. In the latter cases, it can be harder to see the peripheral halo rim.

- In lighter skin, it tends to be pink to red centrally with a more visible peripheral halo rim that is hypopigmented to light pink.

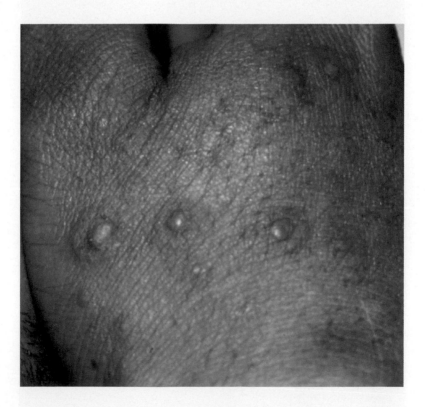

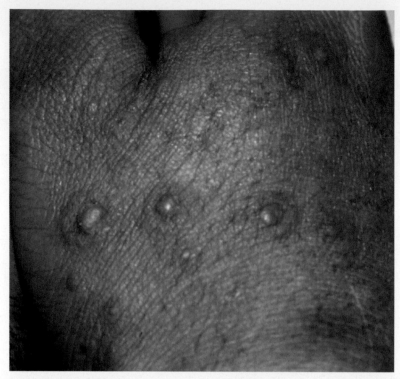

FIGURE 41-1. Pink to violaceous plaques with pink vesicular centers on the dorsal hand. (Reproduced with permission from Wolff K, Johnson RA, Saavedra AP, et al. *Fitzpatrick's Color Atlas and Synopsis of Clinical Dermatology*, 8th ed. New York, NY: McGraw Hill; 2017, Figure 27-38.)

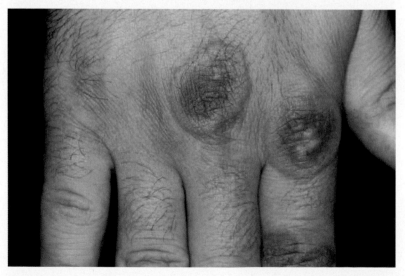

FIGURE 41-2. Targetoid plaques with brighter pink centers exhibiting early vesicular changes and a pale pink rim on the dorsal hand. (Reproduced with permission from Barnhill RL, Crowson AN, Magro CM, et al. *Barnhill's Dermatopathology*, 4th ed. New York, NY: McGraw Hill; 2020, Figure 3-7A.)

Common Cutaneous Disorders in Skin of Color Populations

KEY POINTS

- Sarcoidosis can be the great mimicker and can present with various morphologies and subtypes. It can be mistaken for numerous other conditions including basal and squamous cell carcinoma, lupus, and mycosis fungoides.

- In skin of color, presentations can be pink, violaceous, dark brown, or skin-colored papules and plaques which can have overlying scale. It can also present as hypopigmented patches.

- In lighter skin, it tends to present with a brighter pink to red color and can also be papule, plaque or patch morphology.

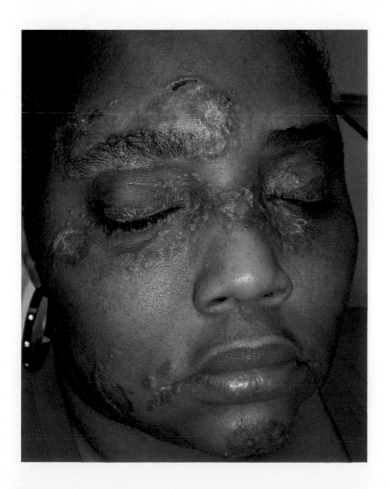

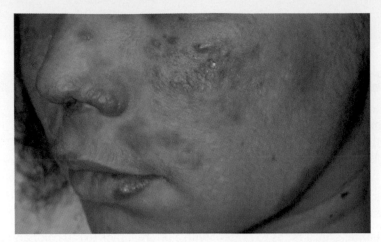

FIGURE 42-1. Deep red to violaceous papules, patches, and plaques along the cheeks, nose, and upper cutaneous and mucosal lips. (From Taylor SC, Kelly AP, Lim HW, et al. *Taylor and Kelly's Dermatology for Skin of Color*, 2nd ed. New York, NY: McGraw Hill; 2016, Figure 74-4. Reproduced with permission from Visual Dx.)

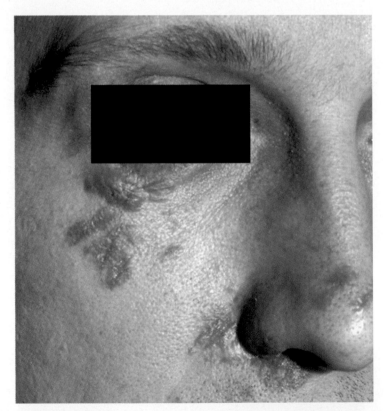

FIGURE 42-2. Orange-brown papules presenting along the lower eyelid, cheek, and nose. Note the lack of scale in this presentation. (Reproduced with permission from Wolff K, Johnson RA, Saavedra AP, et al. *Fitzpatrick's Color Atlas and Synopsis of Clinical Dermatology*, 8th ed. New York, NY: McGraw Hill; 2017, Figure 14-70.)

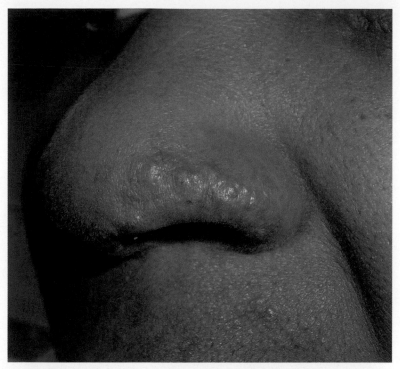

FIGURE 42-3. Fine pink papules coalescing into a plaque along the nasal rim in a Black woman. (From Usatine RP, Smith MA, Mayeaux EJ Jr, et al. *The Color Atlas and Synopsis of Family Medicine*, 3rd ed. New York, NY: McGraw Hill; 2019, Figure 184-2. Reproduced with permission from Richard P. Usatine, MD.)

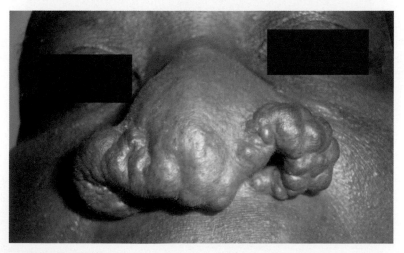

FIGURE 42-4. Clustered papules coalescing into a confluent plaque along the nasal rim and columella. Note the degree of infiltration from these plaques and the disfigurement it is causing to the normal nasal architecture. (From Taylor SC, Kelly AP, Lim HW, et al. *Taylor and Kelly's Dermatology for Skin of Color*, 2nd ed. New York, NY: McGraw Hill; 2016, Figure 95-49. Reproduced with permission from Dr. Anisa Mosam.)

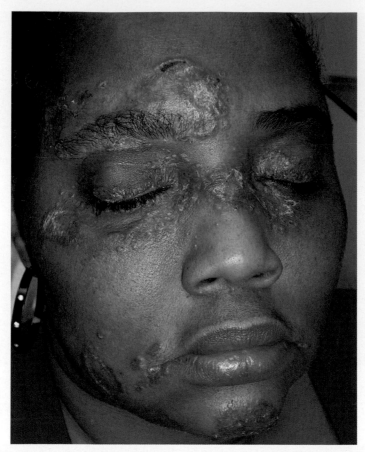

FIGURE 42-5. Pink and violaceous scaly patches and plaques on the face, with increased predominance periocularly and periorally. (From Usatine RP, Smith MA, Mayeaux EJ Jr, et al. *The Color Atlas and Synopsis of Family Medicine*, 3rd ed. New York, NY: McGraw Hill; 2019, Figure 184-13. Reproduced with permission from Richard P. Usatine, MD.)

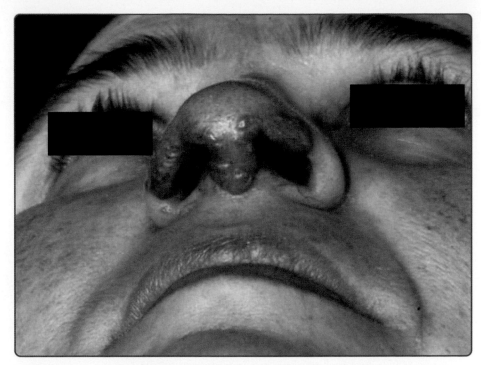

FIGURE 42-6. Bright-red plaques along the inferior nasal ala rim and columella. Note the background erythema on the bilateral cheeks. (Reproduced with permission from Kang S, Amagai M, Bruckner AL, et al. *Fitzpatrick's Dermatology*, 9th ed. New York, NY: McGraw Hill; 2019, Figure 35-7.)

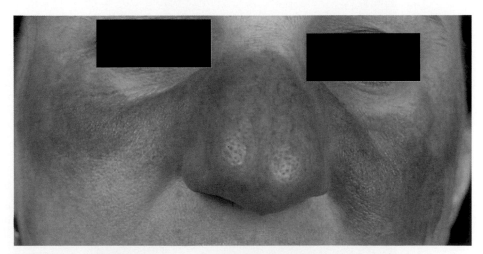

FIGURE 42-7. Pink-purple edematous confluent patch along the nose and medial cheeks. (Reproduced with permission from Desman GT, Barnhill RL. *Barnhill's Dermatopathology Challenge: Self-Assessment & Review.* New York, NY: McGraw Hill; 2016.)

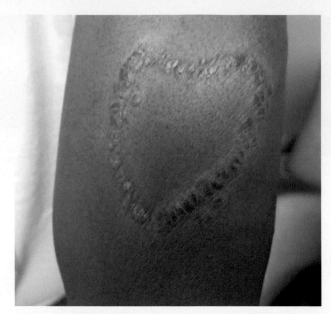

FIGURE 42-8. Brown to pink heart-shaped plaque in the distribution of a tattoo over the knee. Note the variation in color, which can occur among people with skin of color. (From Usatine RP, Smith MA, Mayeaux EJ Jr, et al. *The Color Atlas and Synopsis of Family Medicine*, 3rd ed. New York, NY: McGraw Hill; 2019, Figure 184-9. Reproduced with permission from Amor Khachemoune, MD.)

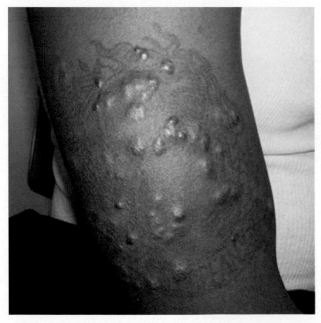

FIGURE 42-9. Bright-red papules and nodules scattered within an upper extremity tattoo. (From Taylor SC, Kelly AP, Lim HW, et al. *Taylor and Kelly's Dermatology for Skin of Color*, 2nd ed. New York, NY: McGraw Hill; 2016, Figure 74-6A. Reproduced with permission from Visual Dx.)

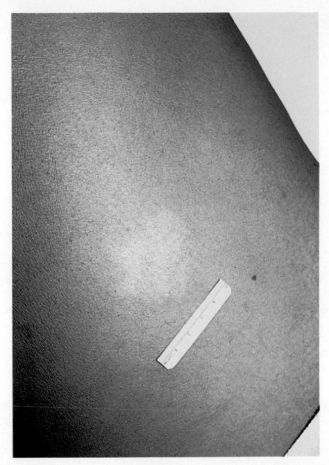

FIGURE 42-10. Discrete hypopigmented patch. (Reproduced with permission from Johnson BL, Moy RL, White GM. *Ethic Skin-Medical and Surgical.* St. Louis, MO: Mosby; 1998.)

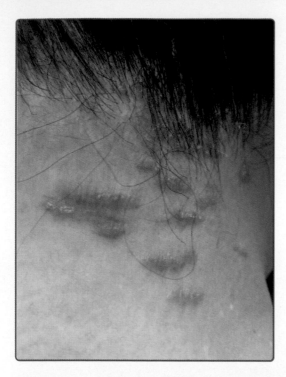

FIGURE 42-11. Linear pink scaly plaques along the posterior neck extending upward into the scalp. (Reproduced with permission from Kang S, Amagai M, Bruckner AL, et al. *Fitzpatrick's Dermatology*, 9th ed. New York, NY: McGraw Hill; 2019, Figure 1-15.)

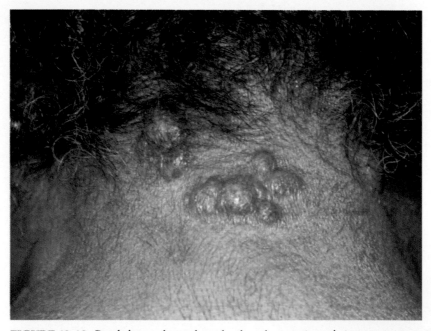

FIGURE 42-12. Purple-brown clustered papules along the posterior neck. (From Taylor SC, Kelly AP, Lim HW, et al. *Taylor and Kelly's Dermatology for Skin of Color*, 2nd ed. New York, NY: McGraw Hill; 2016, Figure 74-10B. Reproduced with permission from Visual Dx.)

KEY POINTS

- Discoid lupus erythematosus (DLE)/Chronic cutaneous lupus (CCLE) can occur in all skin types but has a higher incidence and prevalence in Black individuals.

- In darker skin, it can often present with peripheral dark-brown to violaceus atrophic plaques with central erythema or hypopigmentation. It often also resolves with postinflammatory hyper- or hypopigmentation. This color variation in contrast with baseline pigmentation can be very disfiguring.

- In lighter skin, it tends to present more with hypopigmented to depigmented pink patches.

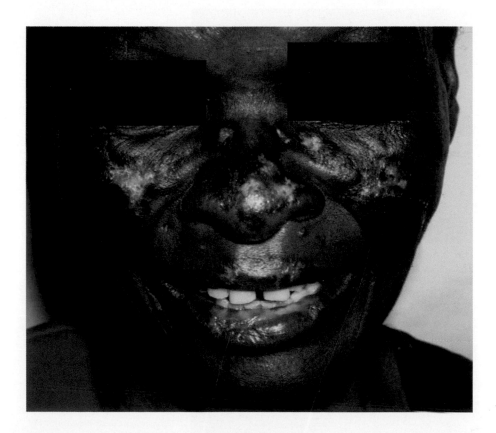

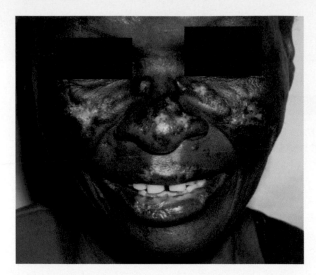

FIGURE 43-1. Dark-black patches and plaques with central erythema on the mid-face of a dark-skinned woman. (From Taylor SC, Kelly AP, Lim HW, et al. *Taylor and Kelly's Dermatology for Skin of Color*, 2nd ed. New York, NY: McGraw Hill; 2016, Figure 95-43. Reproduced with permission from Barbara Leppard.)

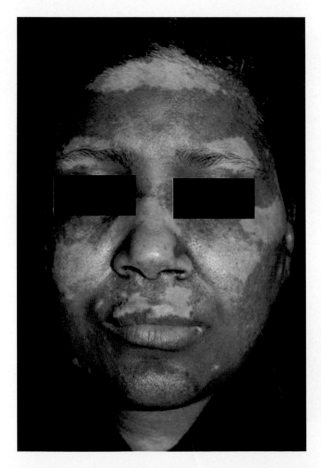

FIGURE 43-2. Hypopigmented patches on the face of a Vietnamese woman secondary to DLE. Note the brighter pink patch along the mid-upper cutaneous lip, signifying areas of active disease. (Reproduced with permission from Wolff K, Johnson RA, Saavedra AP, et al. *Fitzpatrick's Color Atlas and Synopsis of Clinical Dermatology*, 8th ed. New York, NY: McGraw Hill; 2017, Figure 13-16.)

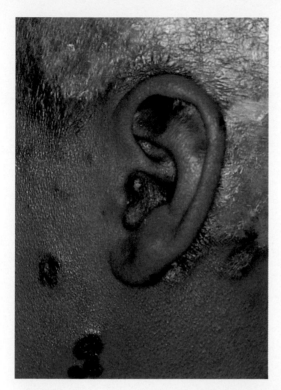

FIGURE 43-3. Black plaques on the face and ear, which also has notable follicular plugging. Along the scalp are visible pink and brown plaques with a periphery of black pigmentation. This is a dark-skinned person with chronic untreated disease. (Reproduced with permission from Kang S, Amagai M, Bruckner AL, et al. *Fitzpatrick's Dermatology*, 9th ed. New York, NY: McGraw Hill; 2019, Figure 61-8A.)

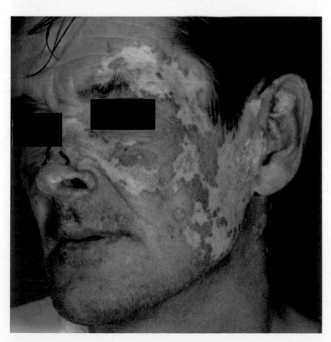

FIGURE 43-4. Depigmented patches with central bright-pink scaly patches on the face, neck, and ear of a lighter-skinned man. (Reproduced with permission from Soutor C, Hordinsky MK. *Clinical Dermatology*. New York, NY: McGraw Hill; 2013, Figure 21-5.)

KEY POINTS

- Vasculitis can present with palpable purpura, which in lighter skin can be bright red to purple but in darker skin can be violaceous to purple-brown.

- In both light and dark skin, there can also be a bullous morphology variant.

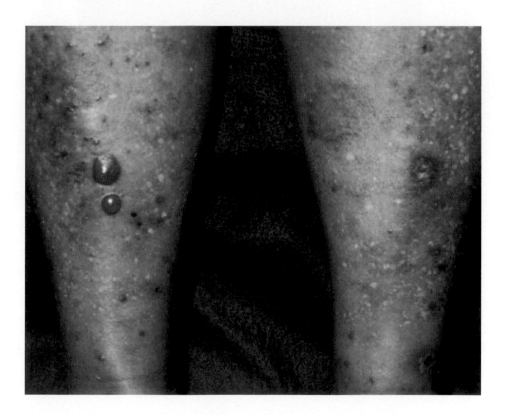

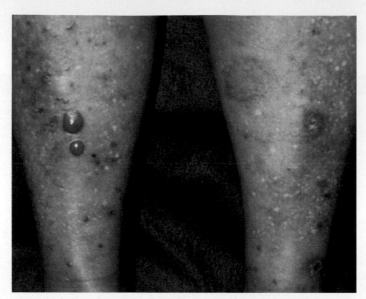

FIGURE 44-1. Purpuric macules and patches with areas of overlying bullae representing bullous leukocytoclastic vasculitis in a person with dark skin. Note also on the distal left extremity the violaceous plaques with a rim of erythema and central erosion. (From Taylor SC, Kelly AP, Lim HW, et al. *Taylor and Kelly's Dermatology for Skin of Color*, 2nd ed. New York, NY: McGraw Hill; 2016, Figure 35-12. Reproduced with permission from William D. James, MD.)

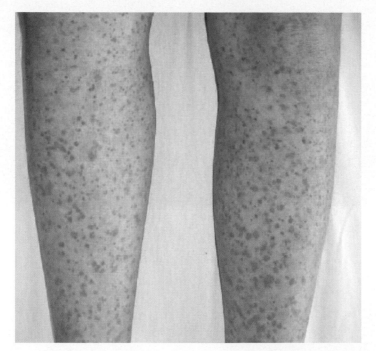

FIGURE 44-2. Densely scattered pink macules and patches along the shin representing a small vessel vasculitis. (From Ali A. *McGraw-Hill Education Specialty Board Review Dermatology: A Pictorial Review*, 3rd ed. New York, NY: McGraw Hill; 2015, Figure 15-7. Reproduced with permission from Dr. Denise Metry.)

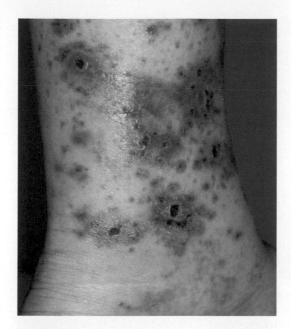

FIGURE 44-3. Red to violaceous macules and superficial plaques with central erosion densely scattered along the lateral lower extremity representing leukocytoclastic vasculitis. (Reproduced with permission from Barnhill RL, Crowson AN, Magro CM, et al. *Barnhill's Dermatopathology*, 4th ed. New York, NY: McGraw Hill; 2020, Figure 9-4A.)

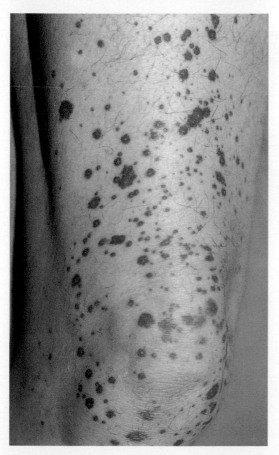

FIGURE 44-4. Palpable purpura. (Reproduced with permission from Soutor C, Hordinsky MK. *Clinical Dermatology*. New York, NY: McGraw Hill; 2013, Figure 25-4.)

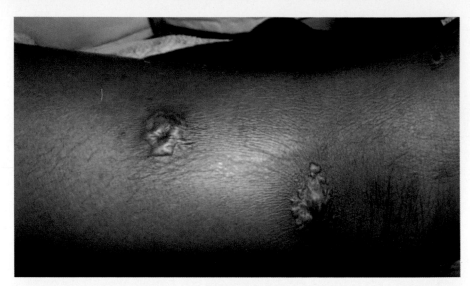

FIGURE 44-5. Violaceous to black bullae surrounded by dusky red erythema on the lower extremity of a person with systemic vasculitis. (Reproduced with permission from Kang S, Amagai M, Bruckner AL, et al. *Fitzpatrick's Dermatology*, 9th ed. New York, NY: McGraw Hill; 2019, Figure 139-3B.)

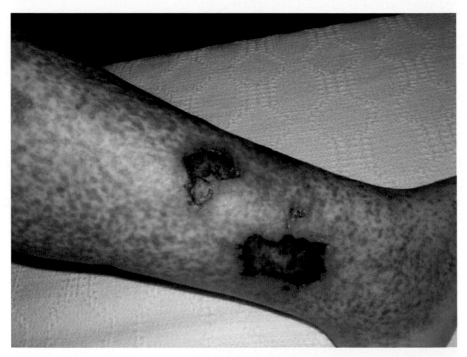

FIGURE 44-6. Superficial ulcers with purple border and surrounding pink-purple erythema. (Reproduced with permission from Kang S, Amagai M, Bruckner AL, et al. *Fitzpatrick's Dermatology*, 9th ed. New York, NY: McGraw Hill; 2019, Figure 139-3C.)

KEY POINTS

- Diabetes mellitus (DM) can have various cutaneous manifestations, which include acanthosis nigricans, necrobiosis lipoidica diabeticorum (NLD), and diabetic dermopathy.

- Acanthosis nigricans (AN) is commonly seen on the neck and intertriginous sites and presents with velvety lichenified plaques that can be accompanied by acrochordons. In lighter skin, AN can be tan to dark brown, and in darker skin, it can be dark brown to black.

- NLD presents with atrophic patches on the shins, which in lighter skin can be brawny to pink-brown, while in darker skin, they tend to be orange-yellow. It can also have underlying vasculature and background erythema, which is often less visible in darker skin.

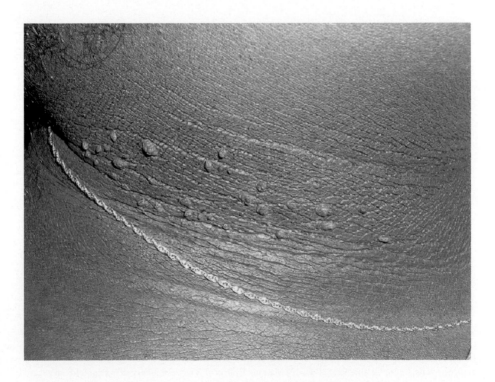

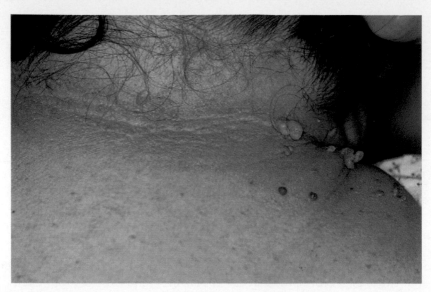

FIGURE 45-1. Light-brown velvety plaque with background erythema and overlying pink and dark-brown acrochordons and seborrheic keratoses, respectively. (From Taylor SC, Kelly AP, Lim HW, et al. *Taylor and Kelly's Dermatology for Skin of Color*, 2nd ed. New York, NY: McGraw Hill; 2016, Figure 68-9. Reproduced with permission from Visual Dx.)

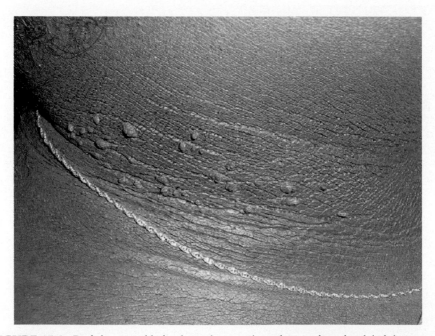

FIGURE 45-2. Dark-brown to black velvety plaque with overlying pedunculated dark-brown acrochordons. (From Usatine RP, Smith MA, Mayeaux EJ Jr, et al. *The Color Atlas and Synopsis of Family Medicine*, 3rd ed. New York, NY: McGraw Hill; 2019, Figure 228-4. Reproduced with permission from Richard P. Usatine, MD.)

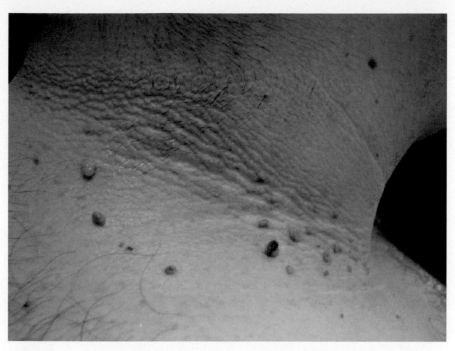

FIGURE 45-3. Velvety thickened tan plaque along the lateral neck with overlying and adjacent skin-colored acrochordons. (From Ali A. *McGraw-Hill Education Specialty Board Review Dermatology: A Pictorial Review*, 3rd ed. New York, NY: McGraw Hill; 2015, Figure 23-8. Reproduced with permission from Dr. Asra Ali.)

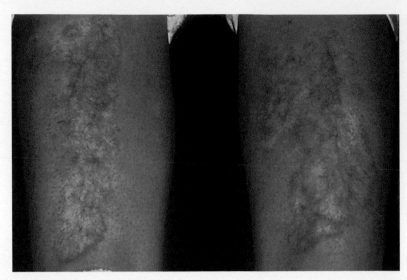

FIGURE 45-4. Yellow-brown atrophic and hypopigmented waxy plaques with subtle visible vasculature on the bilateral anterior shins. (Reproduced with permission from Kane KS, Nambudiri VE, Stratigos AJ. *Color Atlas & Synopsis of Pediatric Dermatology*, 3rd ed. New York, NY: McGraw Hill; 2017, Figure 18-2.)

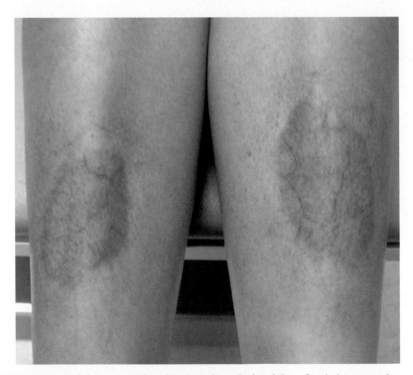

FIGURE 45-5. Pink-brown atrophic plaques with marked visibility of underlying vasculature and background erythema. (From Usatine RP, Smith MA, Mayeaux EJ Jr, et al. *The Color Atlas and Synopsis of Family Medicine*, 3rd ed. New York, NY: McGraw Hill; 2019, Figure 231-1. Reproduced with permission from Suraj Reddy, MD.)

Benign Skin Findings

KEY POINTS

- Striae distensae are vertical atrophic scars that can vary in presentation across skin colors.

- Striae rubra are more common in lighter skin, while striae alba are more common in darker skin.

- Striae rubra tend to present as pink to dark red, while striae alba are hypopigmented to white.

- In darker skin, striae can also be violaceous initially and can resolve as hypopigmented to white over time.

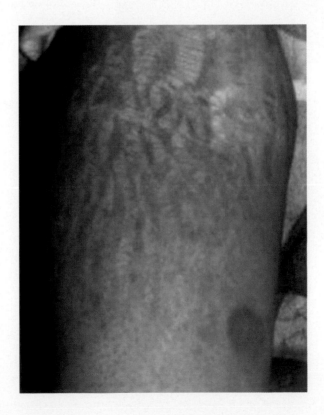

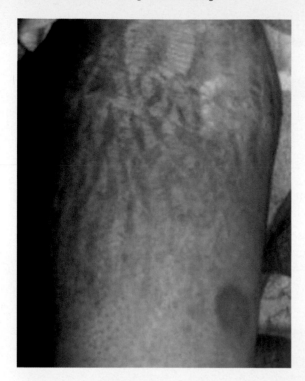

FIGURE 46-1. Dark-brown linear atrophic plaques representing striae distensae in a person with dark skin. (Reproduced with permission from Prose NS, Kristal L. *Weinberg's Color Atlas of Pediatric Dermatology*, 5th ed. New York, NY: McGraw Hill; 2017, Figure 20-21.)

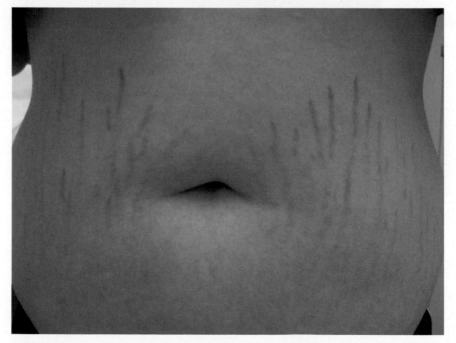

FIGURE 46-2. Linear pink patches on the abdomen of a light-skinned person, representing striae rubra. (Reproduced with permission from Tannous Z, Avram MM, Tsao S, et al. *Color Atlas of Cosmetic Dermatology*, 2nd ed. New York, NY: McGraw Hill; 2011, Figure 60-3.)

KEY POINTS

- Extrinsic and intrinsic aging can vary across racial and ethnic populations.

- In lighter skin, signs of aging include facial volume loss, rhytides, seborrheic keratoses, and photodamage including solar lentigines and mottled pigmentation.

- In darker skin, volume loss and rhytides tend to occur at more advanced ages. Other components of aging in darker skin include the development of dermatosis papulosis nigra, seborrheic keratoses, idiopathic guttate hypopigmentation, and maturational dyschromia.

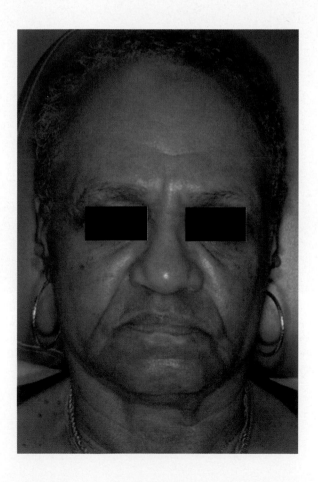

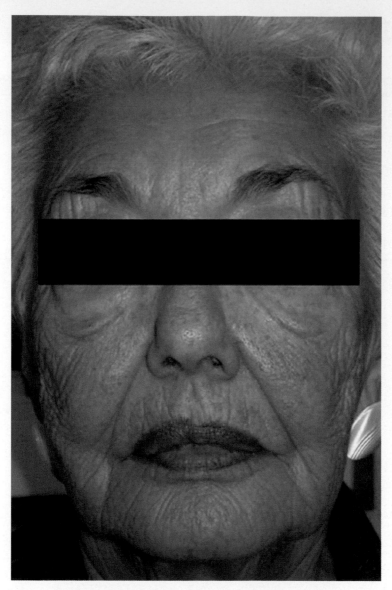

FIGURE 47-1. Facial rhytides, both superficial and deep, which are more prominent periorally along with facial lentigines, superficial telangiectasias, and infraorbital hollowing, with loss of skin elasticity in a woman with lighter skin. Also note the deeper prominence of her nasolabial folds and marionette lines. (Reproduced with permission from Alam M, Bhatia AC, Kundu RV, et al. *Cosmetic Dermatology for Skin of Color.* New York, NY: McGraw Hill; 2009, Figure 9-2A.)

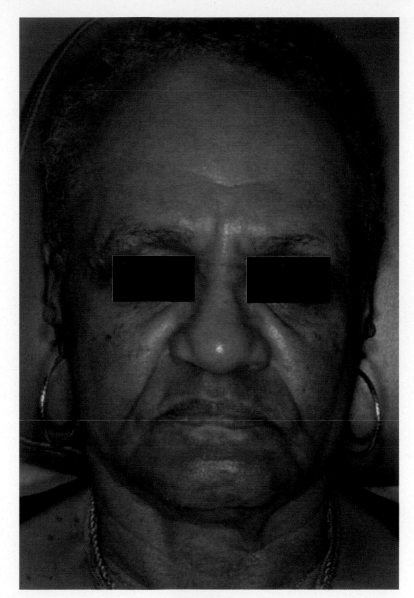

FIGURE 47-2. Superficial and deep rhytides, including prominent nasolabial folds and glabellar and marionette lines in a Black woman. Note also the loss of mid-face volume with infraorbital hollowing. (Reproduced with permission from Avram MR, Avram MM, Ratner D. *Procedural Dermatology*. New York, NY: McGraw Hill; 2015, Figure 58-5.)

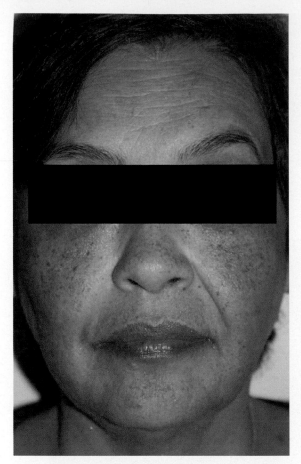

FIGURE 47-3. In contrast, the signs of aging visible in this Asian woman include facial lentigines, superficial rhytides, and less prominent nasolabial folds. (Reproduced with permission from Alam M, Bhatia AC, Kundu RV, et al. *Cosmetic Dermatology for Skin of Color.* New York, NY: McGraw Hill; 2009, Figure 9-2B.)

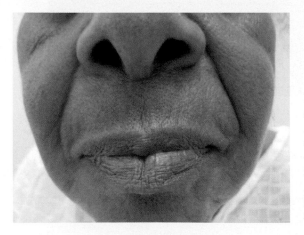

FIGURE 47-4. Prominent nasolabial folds in an elderly African American woman with loss of mid-face volume. (Reproduced with permission from Taylor SC, Kelly AP, Lim HW, et al. *Taylor and Kelly's Dermatology for Skin of Color,* 2nd ed. New York, NY: McGraw Hill; 2016, Figure 19-1.)

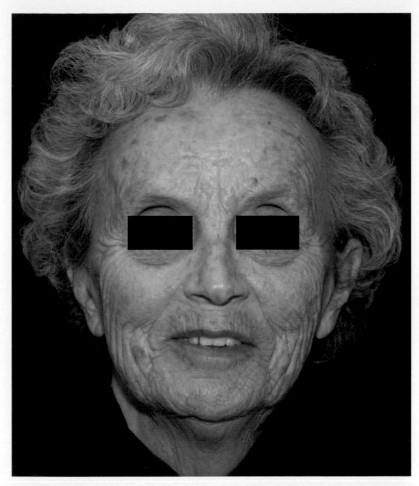

FIGURE 47-5. Facial lentigines, seborrheic keratosis, and superficial and deep rhytides are visible, along with infraorbital hollowing. Note sagging of the skin secondary to loss of elasticity. (Reproduced with permission from Tannous Z, Avram MM, Tsao S, et al. *Color Atlas of Cosmetic Dermatology*, 2nd ed. New York, NY: McGraw Hill; 2011, Figure 1-4A.)

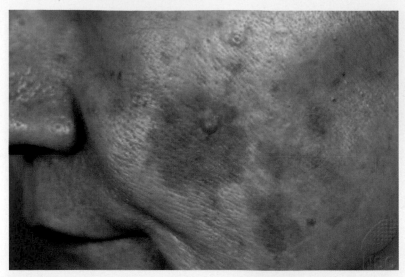

FIGURE 47-6. Large, flat, light-brown patches and papules consistent with pigmented seborrheic keratoses on a background of skin with fine wrinkles in a Chinese person. (From Taylor SC, Kelly AP, Lim HW, et al. *Taylor and Kelly's Dermatology for Skin of Color*, 2nd ed. New York, NY: McGraw Hill; 2016, Figure 77-3B. Reproduced with permission from the National Skin Centre, Singapore.)

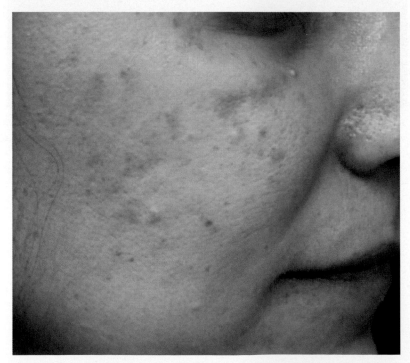

FIGURE 47-7. Southeast Asian woman with light-brown macules on the cheek consistent with facial lentigines. (Reproduced with permission from Taylor SC, Kelly AP, Lim HW, et al. *Taylor and Kelly's Dermatology for Skin of Color*, 2nd ed. New York, NY: McGraw Hill; 2016, Figure 87-4.)

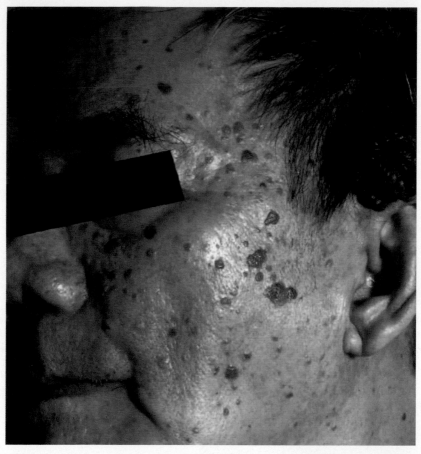

FIGURE 47-8. Numerous dark-brown seborrheic keratoses on a background of facial skin with fine rhytides in a Chinese man. (From Taylor SC, Kelly AP, Lim HW, et al. *Taylor and Kelly's Dermatology for Skin of Color*, 2nd ed. New York, NY: McGraw Hill; 2016, Figure 77-3A. Reproduced with permission from the National Skin Centre, Singapore.)

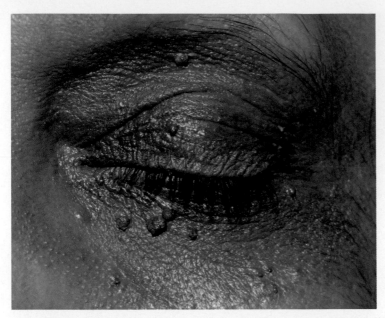

FIGURE 47-9. Periorbital hyperpigmentation with overlying dermatosis papulosis nigra on the upper and lower eyelid. (From Taylor SC, Kelly AP, Lim HW, et al. *Taylor and Kelly's Dermatology for Skin of Color,* 2nd ed. New York, NY: McGraw Hill; 2016, Figure 77-1. Reproduced with permission from the National Skin Centre, Singapore.)

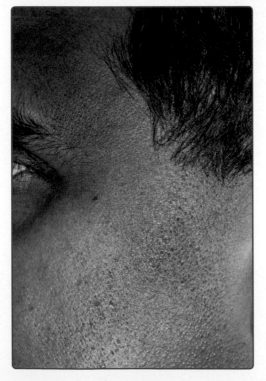

FIGURE 47-10. Dark-brown patch consistent with maturational dyschromia, visible along the preauricular cheek and temple in an Indian man. (Reproduced with permission from Kang S, Amagai M, Bruckner AL, et al. *Fitzpatrick's Dermatology,* 9th ed. New York, NY: McGraw Hill; 2019, Figure 77-8.)

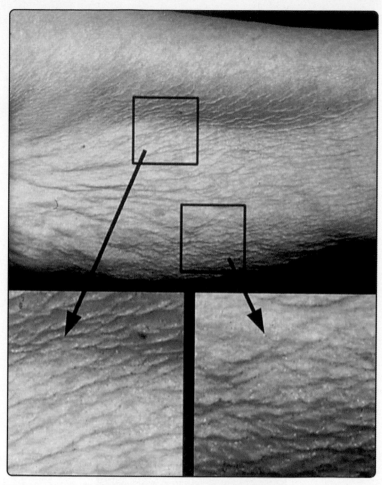

FIGURE 47-11. Fine wrinkling on the ventral upper extremity demonstrating intrinsic aging in an individual with lighter skin. (Reproduced with permission from Kang S, Amagai M, Bruckner AL, et al. *Fitzpatrick's Dermatology*, 9th ed. New York, NY: McGraw Hill; 2019, Figure 106-3.)

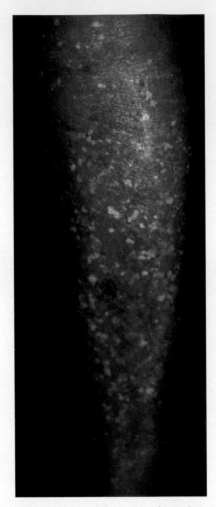

FIGURE 47-12. Densely scattered hypo- and depigmented macules on the anterior shin. (Reproduced with permission from Taylor SC, Kelly AP, Lim HW, et al. *Taylor and Kelly's Dermatology for Skin of Color*, 2nd ed. New York, NY: McGraw Hill; 2016, Figure 20-13.)

Index

Note: Page numbers followed by *f* indicate figures.

A

Acanthosis nigricans, 293, 294*f*–295*f*
Acne
  atrophic scarring in, 145*f*
  chronic changes in, 146*f*–147*f*
  comedones in, 144*f*, 149*f*
  cysts in, 146*f*
  erythema in, 146*f*–147*f*
  hyperpigmentation in, 144*f*
  icepick scarring in, 148*f*, 150*f*
  on lighter vs. darker skin, 143
  macules in, 145*f*, 149*f*–150*f*
  papules in, 145*f*–148*f*
  PIPA in, 242*f*
  pustules in, 145*f*–146*f*
Acne fulminans, 197*f*
Acne keloidalis nuchae
  keloids in, 179*f*–180*f*
  on lighter vs. darker skin, 177
  papules in, 178*f*–180*f*
  pustules in, 178*f*
Acrochordons, 294*f*–295*f*
Aging
  facial lentigines in, 302*f*, 304*f*–306*f*
  facial rhytides in, 302*f*–303*f*, 305*f*
  infraorbital hollowing in, 303*f*, 305*f*
  intrinsic, 309*f*
  in lighter vs. darker skin, 301
  macules in, 306*f*, 310*f*
  maturational dyschromia in, 308*f*
  mid-face volume loss in, 303*f*–304*f*
  nasolabial folds in, 303*f*–304*f*
  periorbital hyperpigmentation in, 308*f*
  seborrheic keratoses in, 306*f*–307*f*
Allergic salute, 20*f*
Atopic dermatitis
  chronic, 15*f*, 16*f*, 21*f*, 27*f*
  erythema in, 16*f*, 17*f*, 19*f*, 21*f*
  excoriations in, 12*f*
  on feet, 19*f*
  on hands, 18*f*
  hyperpigmentation in, 24*f*, 26*f*

  in infants and children, 22*f*–24*f*
  lichenification in, 12*f*, 14–15*f*, 26*f*
  on lighter vs. darker skin, 11
  macules in, 12*f*
  on neck, 25*f*, 27*f*
  papules in
    dark-brown gray, 26*f*
    dark-brown scaly, 23*f*
    fine scaly, 25*f*
    hyperpigmented, 13*f*, 15*f*
    lichenified, 15*f*, 19*f*, 23*f*
    nummular bright-red, 17*f*
    periorbital, 21*f*
    pink and brown, 23*f*
    pink-red, 19*f*
    pinpoint, 13*f*
    red and orange, 22*f*
    red scaly, 26*f*
    skin-colored, 13*f*, 26*f*
  patches in
    hyperpigmented confluent, 15*f*
    hyperpigmented diffuse, 17*f*
    hypopigmented, 24*f*
    lichenified hyperpigmented,
      12*f*, 16*f*
    lichenified pink, 14*f*, 15*f*, 19*f*, 23*f*
    lichenified scaly, 23*f*
    perioral, 22*f*
  periorbital edema in, 20*f*–21*f*
  PIPA in, 241*f*
  plaques in
    dark-brown scaly, 23*f*
    dark-brown thickened, 27*f*
    hyperpigmented, 12*f*, 17*f*
    lichenified, 12*f*, 16*f*, 18*f*, 23*f*
    pink, 19*f*
    red, 16*f*
    red and orange, 22*f*
    red with pink, 16*f*, 18*f*, 26*f*
Axilla
  hidradenitis suppurativa on, 169*f*–170*f*
  psoriasis on, 44*f*

B

Balsam of Peru, contact dermatitis from, 52*f*–53*f*

Basal cell carcinoma
on lighter vs. darker skin, 201
nodules in, 203*f*
papule in, 202*f*
patches in, 206*f*
pigmented, 203*f*–204*f*, 206*f*
plaques in, 203*f*–206*f*
squamous cell carcinoma mimicking, 211*f*–212*f*
ulcerated nodular, 202*f*

Bowen disease, 209*f*

Breasts, psoriasis on, 43*f*, 45*f*

Bullae
in erythema multiforme, 273
in SJS/TEN, 269, 272*f*
in vasculitis, 290*f*, 292*f*

Burrows, in scabies, 135*f*, 137*f*

C

Cellulitis
in diabetes, 109*f*
on lighter vs. darker skin, 107
patches in, 108*f*–109*f*
plaque in, 109*f*

Chemical peel, PIPA after, 245*f*

Chromate allergy, contact dermatitis from, 57*f*

Chronic actinic dermatitis
on lighter vs. darker skin, 255
patches in, 256*f*–257*f*
plaques in, 256*f*

Comedones, 144*f*, 149*f*

Condyloma, 121*f*

Contact dermatitis
erythema in, 56*f*, 58*f*
on lighter vs. darker skin, 49
papules and vesicles in, 56*f*, 58*f*
patches in, 51*f*–53*f*, 58*f*–59*f*
perioral, 50*f*
periorbital edema in, 52*f*
plaques in
dark-brown, 51*f*
fuchsia, 52*f*
pink, 54*f*, 57*f*
pink-brown, 53*f*, 54*f*, 57*f*
pink-gray, 55*f*
violaceous, 56*f*

Cutaneous T-cell lymphoma (mycosis fungoides, Sézary syndrome)
erythroderma in, 225*f*
hydroa vacciniforme-like, 226*f*
on lighter vs. darker skin, 219*f*
macules in, 220*f*–221*f*
patches in, 220*f*–224*f*
vs. pityriasis rosea, 223*f*
plaques in, 220*f*, 222*f*, 226*f*
vs. tinea versicolor, 99*f*
tumor stage of, 226*f*
vesicles in, 226*f*

Cysts
in acne, 146*f*
in dermatosis papulosis nigra, 186*f*

D

Dennie-Morgan lines, 20*f*–21*f*

Dermatofibroma
on lighter vs. darker skin, 187
macules in, 189*f*, 191*f*
nodules in, 190*f*
papules in, 188*f*

Dermatofibroma sarcoma protuberans
exophytic tumor in, 192*f*
hyperpigmentation and hypopigmentation in, 192*f*
on lighter vs. darker skin, 187
plaque in, 192*f*–193*f*
protuberant tumor in, 193*f*

Dermatosis papulosis nigra, 183, 308*f*.
See also Seborrheic keratoses

Diabetes mellitus
acrochordons in, 294*f*–295*f*
cutaneous manifestations on lighter vs. darker skin, 293
erythema in, 296*f*
plaques in, 294*f*–296*f*
seborrheic keratoses in, 294*f*

Digits. *See* Hands and fingers

Dimple sign, 189*f*

Discoid lupus erythematosus/chronic cutaneous lupus erythematosus (DLE/CCLE)
hypopigmentation in, 286*f*–287*f*
on lighter vs. darker skin, 285
patches in, 286*f*–287*f*
plaques in, 286*f*–287*f*

Dyschromia, maturational, 308*f*

E

Eczema, nummular, 243*f*
Eczema herpeticum, 128*f*
Elbow, darkening of (normal variant in SOC), 7*f*
Erythema
    in acne, 145*f*–147*f*
    in atopic dermatitis, 19*f*, 21*f*
    in chronic actinic dermatitis, 257*f*
    in contact dermatitis, 56*f*, 58*f*
    in diabetes mellitus, 294*f*, 296*f*
    in DLE/CCLE, 286*f*
    in eczema herpeticum, 128*f*
    in erythema chronicum migrans, 140*f*
    in fixed drug reactions, 267*f*–268*f*
    in folliculitis, 163*f*
    in hidradenitis suppurativa, 169*f*
    in lichen planus, 80*f*
    in melasma, 234*f*
    in morbilliform drug reactions, 262*f*
    in perioral dermatitis, 158*f*–159*f*
    in PLC, 62*f*–63*f*
    in PMLE, 250*f*
    postinflammatory, 241*f*
    in rosacea, 152*f*, 154*f*
    in squamous cell carcinoma, 208*f*
    in syphilis, 116*f*
    in varicella zoster, 130*f*–132*f*
    in vasculitis, 290*f*, 292*f*
Erythema chronicum migrans, 139, 140*f*
Erythema multiforme
    on lighter vs. darker skin, 273
    plaques in, 274*f*
Erythroderma, in Sézary syndrome, 225*f*
Erythrodermic psoriasis, 46*f*
Eyelids
    atopic dermatitis on, 20*f*, 21*f*
    basal cell carcinoma on, 203*f*
    contact dermatitis on, 53*f*
    dermatosis papulosis nigra on, 308*f*
    molluscum on, 124*f*
    sarcoidosis on, 278*f*
    seborrheic dermatitis on, 73*f*, 75*f*
    SJS/TEN on, 271*f*

F

Face. *See also* Eyelids; Neck
    acne on. *See* Acne
    aging changes on. *See* Aging
    atopic dermatitis on, 19*f*–24*f*
    basal cell carcinoma on. *See* Basal cell carcinoma
    chronic actinic dermatitis, 256*f*–257*f*
    contact dermatitis on, 51*f*–53*f*

    cutaneous T-cell lymphoma, 221*f*, 226*f*
    DLE/CCLE on, 286*f*–287*f*
    fixed drug reactions on, 267*f*
    herpes simplex on, 129*f*
    lichen planus on, 85*f*
    melanoma on, 217*f*
    melasma on, 234*f*–237*f*
    molluscum on, 125*f*
    perioral dermatitis on. *See* Perioral dermatitis
    PIPA on, 242*f*, 245*f*
    PMLE on, 250*f*–251*f*
    pseudofolliculitis barbae on. *See*
        Pseudofolliculitis barbae
    psoriasis on, 30*f*
    rosacea on. *See* Rosacea
    sarcoidosis on, 278*f*–281*f*
    seborrheic dermatitis on, 72*f*–73*f*, 75*f*
    SJS/TEN on, 271*f*–272*f*
    squamous cell carcinoma on. *See* Squamous
        cell carcinoma
    syphilis on, 115*f*–116*f*
    tinea versicolor on, 98*f*
    verruca plana on, 118*f*–119*f*
Feet
    atopic dermatitis on, 19*f*
    contact dermatitis on, 58*f*, 59*f*
    lichen planus on, 82*f*
    melanoma on, 214*f*–215*f*
    plantar, brown macules on (normal variant in
        SOC), 5*f*
    syphilis on, 114*f*
Fingers. *See* Hands and fingers; Nails
Fixed drug reactions
    disseminated, 268*f*
    on lighter vs. darker skin, 265
    patches in, 266*f*–268*f*
Folliculitis
    hyperpigmentation in, 162*f*–163*f*
    infectious, 164*f*
    on lighter vs. darker skin, 161
    papules in, 162*f*–165*f*
    pustules in, 165*f*
Formaldehyde, contact dermatitis from, 52*f*–53*f*
Fragrance, contact dermatitis from, 52*f*, 57*f*
Futcher lines, 6*f*

G

Gluteal cleft
    atopic dermatitis on, 17*f*
    hidradenitis suppurativa on, 169*f*
    squamous cell carcinoma on, 209*f*
Guttate psoriasis, 32*f*

H

Hands and fingers. *See also* Nails
  atopic dermatitis on, 14*f*–15*f*, 18*f*
  contact dermatitis on, 57*f*
  erythema multiforme on, 274*f*
  lichen planus on, 84*f*
  melanoma on, 214*f*, 218*f*
  melanonychia on. *See* Melanonychia
  normal variants in SOC
    brown linear creases on palmar surface, 4*f*
    brown punctate keratoses on digits, 4*f*
    light brown linear streak on nail plate, 5*f*
  PMLE on, 254*f*
  psoriasis on, 36*f*–37*f*
  scabies on, 135*f*, 138*f*
  squamous cell carcinoma on, 211*f*
  syphilis on, 112*f*
  verruca vulgaris on, 120*f*
Henna tattoo, contact dermatitis from, 56*f*
Herald patch, in pityriasis rosea,
    65, 67*f*, 69*f*
Herpes simplex
  on lighter vs. darker skin, 127
  vesicles in, 129*f*
Hidradenitis suppurativa
  atrophic scars in, 168*f*
  on axilla, 168*f*–170*f*
  chronic inflammation in, 209*f*
  on lighter vs. darker skin, 167
Hyperpigmentation
  in acne, 144*f*, 148*f*–149*f*
  in atopic dermatitis, 12*f*, 17*f*,
    25*f*, 26*f*
  in dermatofibroma sarcoma protuberans,
    192*f*
  in folliculitis, 162–163*f*
  in lichen planus, 81*f*
  periorbital, 308*f*
  in PIPA, 241*f*–242*f*
  in PMLE, 250*f*
  in pseudofolliculitis barbae, 172*f*
  in scabies, 134*f*
Hypertrophic scars. *See* Scarring,
    hypertrophic
Hypopigmentation
  in DLE/CCLE, 286*f*–287*f*
  in lichen planus, 86*f*
  in PIPA, 240*f*, 243*f*, 245*f*
  in psoriasis, 36*f*, 48*f*
  in sarcoidosis, 283*f*
  in tinea corporis, 105*f*
  in tinea versicolor, 98*f*–99*f*

I

Icepick scarring, 147*f*–148*f*, 150*f*
Infants and children
  atopic dermatitis in, 22*f*–24*f*
  scabies in, 136*f*–137*f*
Infraorbital hollowing, 303*f*, 305*f*
Inverse psoriasis, 44*f*–45*f*
Isothiazolinone, contact dermatitis from, 53*f*

K

Keloids. *See also* Plaques, keloidal
  in acne keloidalis nuchae, 180*f*–181*f*
  on lighter vs. darker skin, 195
  nodules in, 196*f*
  papules and plaques in, 197*f*
  in pseudofolliculitis barbae, 175*f*
Knees
  increased pigmentation on (normal variant in
    SOC), 7*f*
  psoriasis on, 33*f*, 34*f*
Koebnerization, 80*f*, 91*f*

L

Laser treatments, PIPA after,
    244*f*–245*f*
Lentigines, facial, 302*f*, 304*f*–305*f*,
    306*f*
Lichen nitidus
  on lighter vs. darker skin, 89
  papules in, 90*f*–91*f*
Lichen planus
  annular, 86*f*
  follicular, 86*f*
  hyperpigmentation in, 81*f*
  hypertrophic, 87*f*
  hypopigmentation in, 86*f*
  on lighter vs. darker skin, 77
  papules in
    atrophic brown, 86*f*
    black-gray, 84*f*
    brown-pink, 81*f*
    dark-purple–black, 83*f*
    pink flat-topped, 80*f*
    pink-purple, 82*f*, 87*f*
    purple-brown, 85*f*
    purple-white flat-topped, 83*f*
    red-maroon, 79*f*
    red-purple flat-topped, 80*f*
    skin-colored, 86*f*
    violaceous flat-topped, 87*f*
  patches in, 84*f*
  PIPA in, 240*f*

Lichenification
    in atopic dermatitis. *See* Atopic dermatitis
    in chronic actinic dermatitis, 256*f*
    in contact dermatitis, 52*f*–55*f*, 57*f*
    in psoriasis, 33*f*–34*f*, 47*f*
    in Sézary syndrome, 224*f*
Lips
    contact dermatitis on, 50*f*
    molluscum on, 125*f*
    seborrheic dermatitis on, 75*f*
Lower extremities
    cellulitis on, 108*f*–109*f*
    lichen planus on, 86*f*–87*f*
    normal variants in SOC
        increased pigmentation on knees, 7*f*
        linear demarcation of pigmentation on, 6*f*
    PIPA on, 240*f*–241*f*
    psoriasis on, 32*f*, 33*f*
    sarcoidosis on, 282*f*
    squamous cell carcinoma on, 208*f*

M
Macules
    in acne, 145*f*, 149*f*
    in atopic dermatitis, 12*f*
    brown pinpoint on tongue (normal variant in
        SOC), 8*f*
    brown plantar (normal variant in SOC), 5*f*
    in cutaneous T-cell lymphoma, 220*f*–221*f*
    in dermatofibroma, 189*f*, 191*f*
    in facial lentigines, 306*f*
    in folliculitis, 162*f*, 164*f*
    hypopigmented, 310*f*
    in lichen planus, 78*f*
    in morbilliform drug reactions,
        262*f*–263*f*
    with patches in psoriasis, 36*f*
    in PIPA, 241*f*–242*f*
    in pseudofolliculitis barbae, 174*f*, 176*f*
    in seborrheic dermatitis, 72*f*, 75*f*
    in seborrheic keratosis, 185*f*
    in SJS/TEN, 272*f*
    in syphilis, 114*f*
    in vasculitis, 290*f*–291*f*
Marjolin ulcer, 208*f*
Melanoma
    on lighter vs. darker skin, 213
    on nail, 218*f*
    nodules in, 217*f*
    papules in, 217*f*
    patches in, 214*f*–215*f*
    plaque in, 214*f*, 216*f*

Melanonychia, 229, 230*f*–231*f*
Melasma
    distribution of, 233
    on lighter vs. darker skin, 233
    macules in, 235*f*
    patches in, 234*f*–237*f*
Mid-face volume loss, 303*f*–304*f*
Molluscum
    on lighter vs. darker skin, 123
    papules in, 124*f*–125*f*
Morbilliform drug reactions
    on lighter vs. darker skin, 261
    macules in, 262*f*–263*f*
    papules in, 262*f*–263*f*
Mycosis fungoides. *See* Cutaneous T-cell
    lymphoma

N
Nails. *See also* Hands and fingers
    melanoma on, 213, 218*f*
    melanonychia on, 229, 230*f*–231*f*
    normal variants in SOC, 3, 5*f*
    psoriasis on, 36*f*–37*f*
Nasolabial folds, 303*f*–304*f*
Neck. *See also* Face
    atopic dermatitis on, 25*f*, 27*f*
    chronic actinic dermatitis on, 257*f*
    sarcoidosis on, 284*f*
Nickel exposure, contact dermatitis from, 54*f*, 55*f*
Nodules
    in basal cell carcinoma, 203*f*
    in dermatofibroma, 190*f*
    in hidradenitis suppurativa, 168*f*–169*f*
    in keloid, 196*f*
    in melanoma, 217*f*
    in sarcoidosis, 282*f*
    in scabies, 136*f*–137*f*

P
Papules
    in acne, 145*f*–148*f*
    in acne keloidalis nuchae, 178*f*–180*f*
    in atopic dermatitis. *See* Atopic dermatitis,
        papules in
    in basal cell carcinoma, 202*f*
    in condyloma, 121*f*
    in contact dermatitis, 56*f*, 58*f*
    in dermatofibroma, 188*f*
    in eczema herpeticum, 128*f*
    in folliculitis. *See* Folliculitis, papules in
    in keloids, 197*f*
    in lichen nitidus, 90*f*–91*f*

Papules (*Cont.*):
  in lichen planus. *See* Lichen planus,
    papules in
  in melanoma, 217*f*
  in molluscum, 124*f*–125*f*
  in morbilliform drug reactions, 262*f*–263*f*
  perifollicular, 162*f*, 163*f*
  in perioral dermatitis, 158*f*–159*f*
  in PIPA, 241*f*–242*f*
  in pityriasis rosea, 66*f*, 67*f*, 68*f*
  in PLC, 62*f*
  in PMLE, 250*f*, 251*f*–254*f*
  in pseudofolliculitis barbae, 172*f*–174*f*, 176*f*
  in rosacea, 152*f*–153*f*, 155*f*
  in sarcoidosis, 278*f*–279*f*, 282*f*, 284*f*
  in scabies, 134*f*–137*f*
  in seborrheic dermatitis, 72*f*
  in seborrheic keratosis, 184*f*–186*f*
  in SJS/TEN, 270*f*–272*f*
  in squamous cell carcinoma, 212*f*
  in syphilis, 112*f*–113*f*, 115*f*–116*f*
  in verruca plana, 118*f*–119*f*
  in verruca vulgaris, 120*f*
Para-phenylenediamine, contact dermatitis
  from, 51*f*
Patches
  in atopic dermatitis. *See* Atopic dermatitis,
    patches in
  in basal cell carcinoma, 206*f*
  in cellulitis, 108*f*–109*f*
  in contact dermatitis, 51*f*–53*f*, 58*f*–59*f*
  in cutaneous T-cell lymphoma,
    220*f*–224*f*
  in DLE/CCLE, 286*f*–287*f*
  in erythema chronicum migrans, 140*f*
  in fixed drug reactions, 266*f*–268*f*
  in hidradenitis suppurativa, 169*f*–170*f*
  in maturational dyschromia, 308*f*
  in melanoma, 214*f*–215*f*
  in melasma, 234*f*–237*f*
  in nummular eczema, 243*f*
  in PIPA, 241*f*, 243*f*–244*f*
  in pityriasis rosea, 67*f*
  in PLC, 63*f*
  in psoriasis. *See* Psoriasis, patches in
  in rosacea, 155*f*
  in sarcoidosis, 278*f*, 280*f*–281*f*, 283*f*
  in seborrheic dermatitis, 72*f*–75*f*
  in SJS/TEN, 270*f*–272*f*
  in striae rubra, 300*f*
  in tinea corporis, 102*f*–104*f*
  in vasculitis, 290*f*

Perioral dermatitis
  atopic, 22*f*
  contact, 49*f*, 50*f*
  erythema in, 158*f*–159*f*
  in herpes simplex, 129*f*
  on lighter vs. darker skin, 157
  in melasma, 235*f*
  papules in, 158*f*–159*f*
  plaques in, 159*f*
  in sarcoidosis, 280*f*
  seborrheic, 73*f*
  in SJS/TEN, 271*f*–272*f*
  in syphilis, 115*f*
Periorbital edema
  in atopic dermatitis, 20*f*–21*f*
  in contact dermatitis, 52*f*
Pigmented skin. *See* Skin of color (SOC)
PIPA. *See* Postinflammatory pigment alteration
  (PIPA)
Pityriasis lichenoides chronica (PLC), 61,
  61*f*–63*f*
Pityriasis rosea
  classic presentation on lighter skin, 66*f*
  vs. cutaneous T-cell lymphoma, 223*f*
  herald patch in, 67*f*, 69*f*
  on lighter vs. darker skin, 65
  papules in, 67*f*–68*f*
  plaques in, 66*f*–69*f*
Plaque psoriasis. *See* Psoriasis, plaques in
Plaques
  in atopic dermatitis. *See* Atopic dermatitis,
    plaques in
  in basal cell carcinoma, 203*f*–206*f*
  in condyloma, 121*f*
  in contact dermatitis. *See* Contact dermatitis,
    plaques in
  in cutaneous T-cell lymphoma, 220*f*, 222*f*, 226*f*
  in diabetes mellitus, 294*f*–295*f*
  in DLE/CCLE, 286*f*–287*f*
  in erythema chronicum migrans, 140*f*
  in erythema multiforme, 274*f*
  in hidradenitis suppurativa, 169*f*–170*f*
  in hypertrophic scars, 198*f*
  keloidal
    in acne keloidalis nuchae, 179*f*
    in dermatofibroma sarcoma protuberans,
      192*f*, 193*f*
  in keloids, 197*f*
  in lichen planus, 79*f*, 83*f*
  in melanoma, 214*f*, 216*f*
  perioral, 159*f*
  in pityriasis rosea, 66*f*–69*f*

in PMLE, 251*f*–252*f*
in sarcoidosis, 278*f*–282*f*, 284*f*
in scabies, 136*f*, 138*f*
in SJS/TEN, 270*f*
in squamous cell carcinoma, 208*f*–211*f*
in striae distensae, 300*f*
in syphilis, 114*f*–115*f*
in tinea corporis, 103*f*–105*f*
in varicella zoster, 130*f*
in verruca plana, 119*f*
in verruca vulgaris, 120*f*
PLC (pityriasis lichenoides chronica), 61,
    61*f*–63*f*
Poison ivy, contact dermatitis from, 56*f*
Polymorphous light eruption (PMLE)
    erythema in, 250*f*
    on lighter vs. darker skin, 249
    papules in, 251*f*–254*f*
    plaques in, 251*f*–252*f*
    vs. systemic lupus erythematosus, 250*f*
Pomade acne, 144*f*, 149*f*
Postinflammatory pigment alteration (PIPA)
    in acne, 242*f*
    after psoriasis, 240*f*
    in atopic dermatitis, 241*f*
    erythema in, 240*f*
    hyperpigmentation in, 241*f*–242*f*
    hypopigmentation in, 240*f*, 245*f*
    in lichen planus, 240*f*
    on lighter vs. darker skin, 239
    papules in, 240*f*
    patches in, 240*f*–241*f*, 243*f*–244*f*
Pseudofolliculitis barbae
    hyperpigmentation in, 172*f*
    keloids in, 175*f*
    on lighter vs. darker skin, 171
    macules in, 174*f*, 176*f*
    papules in, 172*f*–174*f*, 176*f*
Psoriasis
    erythrodermic, 46*f*
    guttate, 32*f*
    inverse, 44*f*–45*f*
    on lighter vs. darker skin, 29
    patches in
        dark brown, 44*f*
        hypopigmented, 48*f*
        with macules, 42*f*
        with overlying pustules, 42*f*
        pink-red lichenified, 47*f*
    PIPA after, 240*f*
    plaques in
        annular gray, 30*f*

        bright pink, 33*f*, 37*f*–39*f*, 44*f*
        with crusted pustules, 43*f*
        dark-brown, 48*f*
        light pink, 31*f*, 32*f*
        pink-brown scaly, 40*f*
        pink hyperkeratotic, 36*f*
        pink-red, 30*f*, 31*f*
        pink smooth, 45*f*
        pink with overlying brown pigmentation,
            35*f*
        pink with overlying scale, 34*f*,
            47*f*
        red, 39*f*
        salmon-pink, 37*f*, 41*f*
        silvery-white, 33*f*
        of variegated colors, 36*f*
        violaceous and dark-brown–gray, 32*f*, 33*f*,
            44*f*
        violaceous scaly, 38*f*, 40*f*–41*f*, 47*f*
        violaceous smooth, 45*f*
    pustular, 42*f*–43*f*, 46*f*
Purpura, in vasculitis, 289, 291*f*
Pustules
    in acne, 145*f*–146*f*
    in acne keloidalis nuchae, 178*f*
    in folliculitis, 165*f*
    in psoriasis, 42*f*–43*f*, 46*f*
    in rosacea, 153*f*

R
Rhytides, facial, 302*f*–303*f*, 305*f*, 307*f*
Rosacea
    erythema in, 152*f*, 154*f*
    on lighter vs. darker skin, 151
    papules in, 152*f*–153*f*, 155*f*
    patches in, 155*f*
    pustules in, 153*f*

S
Sarcoidosis
    hypopigmentation in, 283*f*
    on lighter vs. darker skin, 277
    nodules in, 282*f*
    papules in, 278*f*–279*f*, 282*f*, 284*f*
    patches in, 278*f*, 280*f*–281*f*, 283*f*
    plaques in, 278*f*–282*f*, 284*f*
Scabies
    crusted, 138*f*
    hyperpigmentation in, 134*f*
    on lighter vs. darker skin, 133
    papules in, 134*f*–137*f*
    plaques in, 136*f*

Scalp
  acne keloidalis nuchae on, 178*f*–179*f*
  actinic dermatitis on, 256*f*
  basal cell carcinoma on, 206*f*
  DLE/CCLE on, 287*f*
  psoriasis on, 30*f*–31*f*
  sarcoidosis on, 284*f*
  squamous cell carcinoma on, 211*f*
Scarring
  atrophic
    in acne, 145*f*
    in hidradenitis suppurativa, 168*f*
  hypertrophic
    on lighter vs. darker skin, 195
    plaques in, 198*f*
  icepick, in acne, 147*f*–148*f*, 150*f*
  keloid. *See* Keloids
Seborrheic dermatitis
  on lighter vs. darker skin, 71
  papules and macules in, 74*f*
  patches in, 72*f*–75*f*
Seborrheic keratoses
  dark-brown, 307*f*
  in diabetes mellitus, 294*f*–295*f*
  light-brown, 306*f*
  on lighter vs. darker skin, 183
  papules in, 184*f*–186*f*
  patches in, 306*f*
Sézary syndrome, 224*f*–225*f*. *See also*
      Cutaneous T-cell lymphoma
Shoes, contact dermatitis from, 58*f*
Skin of color (SOC), normal variants
      in, 3
  on lower extremities, 6*f*–7*f*
  on nail plate, 4*f*
  on palms, 3*f*
  on plantar feet, 5*f*
  on tongue, 8*f*
  on upper extremities, 7*f*
Squamous cell carcinoma
  erythema in, 208*f*
  exophytic mass in, 212*f*
  on lighter vs. darker skin, 207
  plaques in, 208*f*–211*f*
Stevens-Johnson syndrome/toxic epidermal
      necrolysis (SJS/TEN)
  bullae in, 272*f*
  on lighter vs. darker skin, 269
  macules in, 272*f*
  papules in, 270*f*–272*f*
  patches in, 270*f*–272*f*
  plaques in, 270*f*

Streaks
  in melanonychia, 230*f*–231*f*
  in PIPA, 245*f*
Striae distensae
  atrophic plaques in, 300*f*
  on lighter vs. darker skin, 299
  patches in (striae rubra), 300*f*
Syphilis
  on lighter vs. darker skin, 111
  macules and patches in, 114*f*
  papules in, 112*f*–113*f*, 116*f*
  plaques in, 115*f*

T
Tinea corporis
  hypopigmentation in, 105*f*
  on lighter vs. darker skin, 101
  patches in, 102*f*–104*f*
  plaques in, 103*f*–105*f*
Tinea incognito, 102*f*
Tinea versicolor
  on chin and jawline, 98*f*
  hypopigmentation in, 99*f*
  on light skin, 96*f*, 97*f*
  on lighter vs. darker skin, 95
  macules in, 96*f*–99*f*
  patches in, 96*f*, 99*f*
Tongue, macules on (normal variant in SOC),
      8*f*
Toxic epidermal necrolysis (TEN). *See* Stevens-
      Johnson syndrome/toxic epidermal
      necrolysis (SJS/TEN)
Trunk
  condyloma on, 121*f*
  contact dermatitis on, 54*f*, 55*f*
  cutaneous T-cell lymphoma on, 222*f*–225*f*
  fixed drug reactions on, 266*f*–268*f*
  folliculitis on, 162*f*–165*f*
  melanoma on, 216*f*
  PIPA on, 243*f*–244*f*
  psoriasis on, 38*f*–41*f*, 43*f*, 46*f*, 48*f*
  seborrheic dermatitis on, 74*f*
  SJS/TEN on, 270*f*
  syphilis on, 113*f*
  tinea corporis on, 102*f*–104*f*
  tinea versicolor on, 96*f*–97*f*

U
Ulceration
  in basal cell carcinoma, 201, 202*f*–203*f*, 205*f*
  in cutaneous T-cell lymphoma, 226*f*
  in hidradenitis suppurativa, 169*f*–170*f*

in melanoma, 214f
in squamous cell carcinoma, 207, 208f–209f
in vasculitis, 292f
Upper extremities
cellulitis on, 109f
contact dermatitis on, 56f
cutaneous T-cell lymphoma on, 220f, 223f
darkening of extensor elbow (normal variant
in SOC), 7f
intrinsic aging in, 309f
lichen planus on, 81f
PMLE on, 251f–254f
psoriasis on, 32f, 33f, 42f
sarcoidosis on, 282f
squamous cell carcinoma, 209f–210f
verruca plana on, 118f
verruca vulgaris on, 120f

V
Varicella zoster
on lighter vs. darker skin, 127
vesicles in, 130f–132f

Vasculitis
bullae in, 290f
on lighter vs. darker skin, 289
macules in, 290f–291f
patches in, 290f
plaques in, 291f
purpura in, 291f
Verruca
on lighter vs. darker skin, 117
plana, 118f–119f
squamous cell carcinoma mimicking,
211f
vulgaris, 120f
Vesicles
in cutaneous T-cell lymphoma, 226f
in erythema multiforme, 274f
in herpes simplex, 129f
in scabies, 135f
in varicella zoster, 130f–132f
Vitiligo
vs. cutaneous T-cell lymphoma, 220f
vs. tinea versicolor, 99f